Haematemesis

or

*How One Man Overcame a Fear of Things Medical
and Learned to Navigate His Way Around Hospital*

HENRY G. SHEPPARD

Expanded Third Edition

Copyright © 2016, 2017, 2018 Henry G. Sheppard

All rights reserved.

ISBN: 10 1986007421
ISBN: 13 9781986007429

Haematemesis

*How One Man Overcame a Fear of Things Medical
and Learned to Navigate His Way Around Hospital*

Expanded Third Edition

A merry heart doeth good like a medicine: but a broken spirit drieth the bones. Proverbs 17:2 (KJV)

PHOTOS:
- The photo on the front cover is of the old Royal Adelaide Hospital, taken from Paxton Walk. © Henry G. Sheppard 2017.
- The photo on the back cover was taken at *The Elephant* British pub at a lunch to celebrate the author's sixty-third birthday. *Ten years of leukaemia and still doing lunch*! © Henry G. Sheppard 2017.

Contents

Dedication 7
Haematemesis 9
Foreword to the Third Edition 11
Foreword to the Second Edition 13
Foreword to the First Edition 15
Chapter 1 - *Thinking of England* 17
Chapter 2 - *The Bubble-in-the-Middle* 19
Chapter 3 - *Patient-Centred Care* 27
Chapter 4 - *Catastrophe and Woe* 35
Chapter 5 - *The White-Knuckle Low Moan* 43
Chapter 6 - *A Bum Virgin* 47
Chapter 7 - *A Season in Prison* 53
Chapter 8 - *The Shrieking Dalek* 63
Chapter 9 - *Clockwork Puppy* 69
Chapter 10 - *Cannibalistic Inhalation* 73
Chapter 11 - *Shove-Head-Bang!* 77
Chapter 12 - *Dead Man Walking* 81
Chapter 13 - *Haematology vs Oncology* 83
Chapter 14 - *Bleeding From the Eyes* 87
Chapter 15 - *The Throat Alien* 97
Chapter 16 - *Do You Have Any Pain?* 103
Chapter 17 - *Glowing in the Dark* 107
Chapter 18 - *Eye of Newt, and Toe of Frog* 113
Chapter 19 - *Dignity, Always Dignity* 117
Chapter 20 - *Curried Egg Sandwich* 121
Chapter 21 - *Baby Octopus* 125

Chapter 22 - *Chimes Ringing Out* 133
Chapter 23 - *The Bloody Toe Saga* 141
Chapter 24 - *The Final Insult* 149
Chapter 25 - *Discharge Against Medical Advice* 157
Chapter 26 - *Robot Walker* 169
Chapter 27 - *Rabbit Stir Fry* 179
Chapter 28 - *The Freckle* 187
Chapter 29 - *Wedge-tailed Eagle* 191
Chapter 30 - *In The Pink* 197
Chapter 31 - *Lessons Learned* 200
INDEX 208

Dedication

To Annette Tiller,
whose encouragement has been unfailing,
and whose invitation to high tea is on a par
with receiving an imperial honour.

Haematemesis

noun: *the vomiting of blood*
Official pronunciation: ˌhē-mə-ˈtem-ə-səs
My pronunciation: hem-mar-tem-are-siz

Origin early 19th century:
from *haemato-* 'of blood' + Greek *emesis* 'vomiting'.

More broadly: *barf, chuck, chunder, disgorge, heave, puke, regurgitate, retch, spew, vomit*
the reflex act of ejecting the contents of the stomach through the mouth

—⊱⊰—

This book relates the journey of a medical innocent through the wilds of the hospital system.

Names have been changed, disguised or ignored altogether in the interests of protecting the guilty and the undecided. The innocent need no protection. Their anonymity herein is a form of collateral damage, of the kind that occurs any time lawyers are suspected of loitering in the undergrowth.

I would like to thank the dozens of unknown blood donors, without whom I wouldn't be here today to write this reliable account of life on the other side of the medical looking glass.

Thank you. Thank you. Thank you. Thank you. Thank you. Thank you.
Thank you. Thank you. Thank you. Thank you. Thank you. Thank you. Thank you.
Thank you. Thank you. Thank you . Thank you. Thank you. Thank you. Thank you.
Thank you. Thank you. Thank you. Thank you. Thank you. Thank you. Thank you. Thank you.
Thank you. Thank you. Thank you. Thank you. Thank you. Thank you. Thank you. Thank you.
Thank you. Thank you. Thank you. Yes, I have too much time on my hands; this is the result. Thank you. Thank you. Thank you.

Foreword to the Third Edition

I have no real excuse for expanding *Haematemesis*, other than the fact that stuff continued to happen to me. The world turned, old buildings were replaced by new, diseases progressed or were joined by others, there were more transfusions, new treatments, a drug trial, and so it went.

I thought I had already run out of body parts to be violated by medical staff, but I was wrong.

This book was pulled together with the assistance of my wife. Herein she is known as "my wife". Around the house she is known as "Wifely", a term often uttered in plaintive tone. Other people call her "Rainee", for that is her name. She finds things I've lost; she remembers things I've forgotten; she anticipates matters of significance and prepares for them; she comforts me silently during those times when I sit in the corner and weep piteously. If she were writing this, she would bang on about cleaning and washing and ironing, things I often take for granted. I am grateful, deeply grateful, and intend to say so more often.

You will see a few names in the book, not many. There are hundreds of others who contributed to my present state of health. I haven't listed them out of a fear of forgetting the ones I most wanted to mention. Please forgive my cowardice.

And so it is, with a sense of mild amazement that I'm still here, I say to you, Gentle Reader, *nostrovia*!

Foreword to the Second Edition

Haematemesis was born out of a flurry of frightening experiences, first recorded in a random series of e-mails to friends, then — following numerous requests from my correspondents — gathered together and supplemented into what became the first edition.

That book travelled.

Most people found it amusing, as had been intended. These pleaded for more: more adventures, more laughs, more descriptions of the denizens of the medical underworld.

A small number hated it and attacked the writer as a sexist / racist / classist / ageist / elitist / deplorable / misogynist fool with an anti-medical agenda. Perhaps they are right. I don't think so, but I don't have the energy to raise a defence. I just wish the haters good health and a long life.

Some of the people who reacted badly to the book had suffered their own cancer scares, with traumatic treatments and bad experiences at the hands of a range of medical personnel. They fail to see anything funny about chemotherapy / radiotherapy / cancer / hospital / nose bleeds / anal probes / catheters / etc. and have yet to come to terms with their ordeal, but we all move at our own pace.

The most common complaint arose from the age-old conflict between English-English and American-English, with some Australian-English variants thrown in. I have made minor changes to some of the wording in order to, hopefully, make my meaning clear to English speakers of all stripes. If in doubt, I went with

Australian-English and a prayer that confused readers have recourse to Google for further clarification.[1]

There were comments about the pop culture references. These appeared spontaneously as I wrote and I saw no reason to delete them. They reflect the world I've lived in all these years.

The best of the responses I received were from strangers who became friends. Their kind comments kept me smiling for days. Thank you, one and all.

When I first published *Haematemesis*, I assumed that my medical adventures were at an end. All that lay ahead of me would be a slow return to normality or a sudden drop off the perch. (I'm an optimist at heart.)

The reality was that the light at the end of the tunnel consisted of new medical problems, more treatments, further horizons to broaden and lessons to learn, new friends to make, new toes to tread upon, and an occasional battle to fight.

I've always found the truth more interesting than the idea that someone might like me better if I kept my mouth shut.

Out of all that came this expanded second edition. There were discussions about publishing a companion book to *Haematemesis*, called *Anastomosis*, but that might have been a book title too far. As it is, many people struggle with *Haematemesis*. I think of it as another example of my sense of humour getting me into trouble. I'm stuck with it now, so let's make the best of things.

Enjoy the book. Share with friends. And keep yourself nice.

---

[1] Where I thought it might help, I added a footnote.

Foreword to the First Edition

While I was in hospital (the first time), my wife — chatting happily with on-duty nurses — told a story from when she was a young student nurse on night shift at a country hospital. A patient began vomiting blood, which I'm assured is a frightening sight and not something I've tried myself. She called for the charge nurse, who instructed her to ring the duty doctor at home. He answered and she stammered out the message she'd been instructed to convey, that the patient was suffering a haematemesis, except she couldn't get that word out. In desperation she finally said, "There's blood everywhere!"

The doctor, irritable at having been roused out of a deep sleep, roared at her: "Haematemesis! Haematemesis! Haematemesis!"

I've associated the word with my experiences ever since.

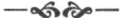

This novel may be thought of as the writer suddenly disgorging some of the fear, hope, pain, confusion and amusement accumulated during his sudden loss of independence and unexpected reliance on men and women in white coats.

The kindness of these wonderful people can never be repaid.

Then, again, there were a few of the other sort...

Chapter One

It all started with the symptoms, of course. Night sweats and endless coughing; the same things that led to my General Practitioner diagnosing the leukaemia in the first place. He did that two weeks after an Ear Nose and Throat surgeon — having conducted a bunch of tests, culminating in a barium swallow[2] — informed me that it was all in my head.

"I can give you the name of a good psychiatrist."

"Thanks, but I'll stick with the leeches for now."

That was back in 2007 and six months of chemotherapy followed. At the end, I had yet another bone marrow biopsy and was declared to be in remission.

Hallelujah!

In 2015, the symptoms returned. I was now out of remission. I dealt with the situation in the time-honoured manner: I went into denial.

I figured that if I ignored it, it would go away.

I hummed *God Save The Queen* under my breath and thought of England. Not that I'd ever been there, but every Australian knows the place well from television. It's a land where the sun shines every day and the Queen takes carriage rides through throngs of

---

[2] A **Barium swallow** involves you swallowing a liquid suspension of barium sulphate before a series of X-rays are taken of your upper digestive tract. Barium is a naturally occurring element that appears white on X-ray.

cheering, flag-waving Poms[3] before lunch. Six white horses up front with a couple of liveried footmen, a couple more at the back, and Prince Phillip sitting up straight, obviously wondering what day it was, but asking Lillibet instead, "What's for lunch?"

We were taught at school that the two liveried footmen at the back of the carriage were equipped with large nets, in case Phil ever escaped the carriage and went walkabout, but I don't know if that's true.

The humming and thinking-of-England delayed the inevitable, but not by much. As the Yanks say, "You can't fight City Hall."

I had previously sworn that I would never undergo the horror of chemotherapy again.

Ever.

I'd lie down in a darkened room and embrace my conclusion, during which time I'd ring down the curtain and join the choir invisible.

Which is all well and good, unless your conclusion remains delayed while you wrestle with your symptoms. Especially the endless coughing.

There comes a point when the neighbours can't take it anymore. The woman over the back fence started shouting abuse every morning while I coughed through breakfast. She was never a nice person, but this was a new low.

Her daily reminders of the impact of my involuntary hacking and hawking started to wear on me. The wheezing and gasping

---

[3] The terms *Pommy*, or *Pom* for short, are slang for someone from England. It is generally believed that "Pommy" originated as a contraction of "pomegranate", Australian rhyming slang for "immigrant".

interfered with phone calls. The rasping and croaking hampered my efforts at murmuring sweet nothings to my wife. My sloppy kisses took on an aerosol quality, which repulsed her.

I had to do something.

I went to see the oncologist, who later turned out to be a haematologist, but that was a confusion for another day. I later came to know him as "Dr. Tease".

He asked about my symptoms, talked about tests (CT scan, bone marrow biopsy), and muttered "chemotherapy" so softly I'm sure he thought I didn't hear him: the subliminal approach to patient management.

I explained that I'd sworn to never do chemo again. He asked the probing question: Why not?

"I didn't enjoy it last time. It was too horrible. No more for me."

I'd laid out the facts in an indisputable manner. Confident that my logic was flawless, my position unassailable, I leaned back in the flimsy plastic chair that tilted to the left, coughed heartily, and awaited his inevitable congratulations over the heroic manner in which I'd dealt with my suffering.

"And that was your *only* problem with chemotherapy?"

In my imagination, I could hear John Cleese asking, in murmured confidential tone, as of a spiritual advisor encouraging the unburdening of one's soul: 'Didn't lose a lung, or a limb, or the sight in one eye, did we? Got all our fingers and toes, have we? No sign of rickets, cleft palate, pigeon chest, spinal dimple, scoliosis, boils, or... jaundice of the back?'

There was a pause: a long, pronounced, emphatic pause that insinuated itself into every corner of the tiny consultation room. I began to feel intimidated.

"Ahh, no. Yes. I mean, it was too horrible."

And surely that was reason enough to justify my refusal. Wasn't it?

He took a break from stroking his chin, placed both hands on the desk, took a deep breath which caused him to inflate in front of me until he assumed the *hauteur* of the scariest school teacher who ever stared me down, then said in a headmasterly voice:

"*Nobody*... enjoys it. It's not meant to be fun."

The implication was indisputable: I was a wimp.

The flimsy plastic chair that tilted to the left was all that kept me from sinking into the floor out of shame. The oncologist took pity on me.

"There have been some developments since you last went through chemo. For instance, there's a tablet version available now."

"No needles?"

"Well, less needles. Some would be intravenous, but most oral."

For the briefest moment, I brightened up. Then he continued, "Trouble is, you did so well last time with the older methods that you don't qualify for the oral drugs."

I couldn't believe it; it had all been a tease.

Chapter Two

The question of chemotherapy was premature, as no one had proven that the leukaemia was back. The obvious next step was testing to establish the facts of the matter.

That meant a CT scan and a bone marrow biopsy.

I was referred to a suburban hospital with pretensions to modernity; its prized asset a bulky white donut, known as a CT scanner. That's a computed tomography scanner to you, or a computerized axial tomography scanner (CAT scanner), if you're feeling flash.

I was eventually shown to a broom closet, with a door at either end. It had a wooden bench on one side, with a pile of old cotton gowns slumped in a heap. I was ordered to strip to the waist from both ends and put on a gown. A quick sift through the pile revealed that they came in two sizes: Too Small and Much Too Small.

Once I closed the door and fitted the two sliding door locks, the latch, and the floor and ceiling bolts, I disrobed, coughed heartily, then wriggled into a Too Small gown. An array of thin cords flapped against my back. I reached for these, but for a long time they eluded my grasp. I'd just captured a midlevel pair when the other door opened and a wisp of a China doll in a white outfit asked, "Ready are we?"

Obviously not. My back was bare, while my pale arse shimmered a shy glance in her direction. She seemed not to notice, but quickly knotted a few of the strings, then led me, like a well-trained giant panda, into a larger place where the CT scanner rested in all its glory.

The white donut had a long metal feeder tray attached, much like the oven conveyer they use at Pizza Hut. The complete assemblage lived in a poorly lit room and would not have looked out of place on the *Millenium Falcon*. I was assisted (pushed) onto the feeder tray and ordered not to move.

The donut gave off a continuous hum, like the engines of the Star Trek *Enterprise*. I waited to hear Scottie on the intercom announcing that the engines couldn't take it anymore, but all I heard was more hum and a small click as the feeder tray shifted an inch, into the starting position.

I braced for the sound of the starter's pistol.

China Doll moved to the next room. The door closed with a clunk and vacuum hiss, as in any good sci-fi film. She bent over a table where she appeared to be making moves in an ongoing holographic chess game against an invisible opponent.

All I could think was, "Let the Wookie win."

The machine spoke to me. It said something about relaxing and not wriggling about quite so much, as if wriggling about were for my amusement rather than a desperate attempt to minimise the discomfort of my position.

I lay pointed, head first, into the donut hole. A search for peace of mind led to me focusing in the other direction. I peered above my girth toward my feet, but in a sunset effect of the nether extremities, they receded from view.

My eyes fixed on the most prominent feature — not necessarily the most fashionable aspect of a mature endomorphic structure — my abdominal equator; the bubble-in-the-middle that tells you I'm on the level; the designer padding that made me popular with people who needed hugs. The longer I looked at it, the more the curve appeared to swell.

My eyes flicked back to the donut hole, which looked to be dangerously narrow and possibly shrinking. I tried to hold the two images in my mind simultaneously, while drawing on the algebraic lessons of youth to compute capacity relative to volume.

If a train carrying a hundred people left Boston at eight ayem...

No, that's not it.

The machine spoke to me again. I expected it to announce the jump to hyperspace, but instead it said, "Take a deep breath and hold it."

I took a deep breath and held it.

I was about to be sucked inside a life-threatening machine, while my broad shoulders, so attractive in youth, sagged over the side of the tray. I tucked my thumbs under my thighs in the hope that my hands wouldn't wave about in a moment of excitement.

The oven conveyer gave another little jump, then dragged me backward. It became a race to tell which would snag first, belly or shoulders.

I pictured Homer Simpson jammed inside the children's water slide for eight hours, while being roundly cursed by every tradesman within shouting distance, and I hoped it would be my shoulders. My chances of attracting sympathy for skeletal issues were greater than those relating to blubber. People can be so unkind about blubber.

By now I had reached the limit of my breath-holding capacity. I'd kept my eyes closed, so as to not witness blood dribbling from the flesh shaved from my gut or oozing from my crushed shoulders. I was feeling fragile and my need to breathe came as a useful distraction.

I released my breath in a slow, smooth exhalation. The conveyer tray clunked to a stop. I expected the machine to tell me I'd done it all wrong and now we would have to do it again, and keep doing it until we got it right.

Then I realised, I'd survived! I'd become the Apollo 13 of the moon program; a short messy trip, but no fatalities. The machine started to speak and my *joie de vivre* evaporated.

"We'll do that again, but this time we're gonna insert a drip in your arm, so we can get some dye in your system. Help us spot irregularities."

China Doll reappeared on my left, armed with needles. I closed my eyes.

"A little prick. Three, two, one. There."

There was the moment of impact, when sharp metal tore through my flesh.

"Might hurt a bit at first, but the moment will pass and you won't feel a thing."

I wanted to ask: "Because of the shock or because of the loss of blood?" but she was already wriggling the needle inside my arm.

"Nahh. Can't get that one in. Let's try the other arm."

She extracted the length of steel, slapped some duct tape over the wound, then moved around the feeder tray.

"Other people have problems getting in your veins?"

"All the time. I did six months of chemo back in 2007 and my veins went into the Witness Protection Program. Now they're living interstate under assumed names."

"Okay then." She raised her voice: "Get Roger."

There came the muffled sound of someone talking on a phone in the room next door. I assumed it was the Wookie.

"Roger's a radiologist. He's the expert," China Doll confided in a voice filled with admiration. "Never misses."

There was a scratching sound, and some snuffling and low growls from next door, then an educated voice announced: "Roger says not to bother. We can go ahead without the dye; the scan we've got will do."

And thus was I introduced to that wonderful arrangement whereby a radiologist gets paid more for a scan with a drip in the arm than a scan without; but time was money and Roger wasn't going to slow the rate at which his money accumulated by wasting time on someone with difficult veins.

So now the fate of my diagnosis would rest on a one-shot scan.

And a bone marrow biopsy.

Chapter Three

The bone marrow biopsy was to take place at the oldest hospital in town, which had been the scene of my first ever biopsy back in the 1970s. In those days, they didn't bother with any anaesthetic, beyond some applied locally for the benefit of the one-eighth of an inch of flesh above the iliac crest; which is to say, the hip bone.

That event occurred with me lying on my side on a stainless-steel table, while a muscular young doctor grunted his way, one by one, through the layers of bone protecting the marrow. The crunching sound he made chilled me to the, ah... bone. Once through, he plunged a needle into the defenceless structure and extracted his fill.

Up to that moment, I had entertained the false belief that there was no feeling inside bones. Ha ha ha. Stupid me. (Ever been kicked in the shins?)

An exquisite pain, quite unlike any other I had experienced, shot through my hip and set up echoes throughout my chest and head. I might have wet myself, I'm not sure. My grip on the side of the stainless steel table tightened sufficiently to leave fingerprints embedded in the metal. Sweat broke out all over and I began to sob softly.

The doctor waltzed from the room, clutching the precious marrow and humming triumphantly. I was left to peel myself from the slab, towel off the sweat, and apply a spare piece of duct tape to the wound.

So, when the time came for me to return to the scene of that particular crime, I did so with no small sense of apprehension.

I shouldn't have worried. Things were different now. We live in the brave new world of patient-centred care, sometimes referred to as Person-Centred Care — the caps add emphasis, which prove they really mean it, while "person" is a kinder, gentler word, bringing with it the promise of better drugs during treatment.

The hospital money people refer to this as "consumer engagement," or "patient participation," or even "citizen engagement," though some of the cynics say it just means more paperwork.

The oncologist decided that, as I am an insulin-dependent diabetic, I should have a pre-op visit with an anaesthetist[4]. I arrived on time for the appointment, only to be told that the visit had been cancelled, as well as the biopsy.

My shocked expression negated any need for discussion.

The young woman on the front desk leapt to the phone to enquire of the officiating party the reason for their action. A long pause gave way to the simple explanation that there was someone else in the system with a similar name, who had cancelled, so my appointment had been deleted.

"Happens all the time," came the smiling observation.

I took no comfort from that and it probably showed on my face. Several nurses had clustered in the vicinity, all intrigued to observe the outworking of any stuff-up that couldn't be traced back to them. "You should complain," said one. "Yeah," chorused some others.

---

[4] *Anaesthetist* is the British/Australian version; the American version is *anaesthesiologist*. These are physicians who deliver medical care to patients needing general or local anaesthesia for surgery and related procedures. Yes, they're doctors, too, and they'd like a little respect.

That surprised me. I would have thought that complaints were bad for everybody. "You're kidding!"

"No. She's done this before. A formal complaint might be what she needs to get her attention."

"Okay. If you say so." I paused, then enlarged on my thinking. "I do have that skill."

They all laughed. I'm not sure why.

The other thing they did was resuscitate my appointments.

I sat with a nurse who laboured through the pages of my medical history, as we together added to and amended the official record. Then I was left sitting in a waiting room, clutching my *bona fides* — a piece of paper with the details of the biopsy which was to take place on the following Tuesday.

Shortly after, I ended up in a small room chatting with an effervescent, if tiny, Chinese doctor, Doctor Le. No, not Lee. Only one E.

"Why waste ink?"

She worked through my notes, read my newest piece of paper and added it to the file, asked a bunch of questions, then enquired of me: "What do you think is the worst thing that could happen to you during the procedure?"

"I could die."

I knew that because my wife — who had had many years of experience as a theatre sister[5] — had told me, oh, hundreds of times.

---

[5] A **theatre sister** In Britain/Australia is an **OR nurse** in the USA.

The doctor was thrilled. She took my answer as evidence of a mature, grounded realism, rather than world-weary fatalism; and superior to the pixie-dust fantasies of the delusional.

"Yes, but I don't think you're going to die."

"Good. Neither do I."

"So," she said, "I'm recommending that your requirements be handled by an anaesthetic clinician. He does an excellent job."

She wrote out her own piece of paper with instructions for handling the crisis that arises when insulin-dependent diabetics stop eating. Most importantly, she confirmed the date of the biopsy, in writing: the following Tuesday.

This all happened on a Wednesday. I idled away the Thursday, then we went to town for shopping and lunch on the Friday. Once we got home, I discovered a message on the phone which talked about a booking for a bone marrow biopsy on the following Monday.

Because this occurred so late, I was unable to ring and clarify the situation. A weekend followed, which also precluded an attempt at clarification.

In the absence of any confirmed facts, I reasoned thus: The Monday appointment was the original, which had been cancelled by accident and presumably been reinstated when the mistake was discovered. The Tuesday appointment had been made and confirmed, in writing, by a nurse and an anaesthetist, and was likely to be the reliable time.

The worst-case scenario for an insulin-dependent diabetic would be that I went through the fasting process, arrived early on Monday morning, only to find that the anaesthetic arrangements put in place by Dr. Le would not be available until Tuesday. Then I would have to go through all that again. Not ideal.

Monday arrived and, still dressed in pyjamas and fluffy slippers, I coughed heartily, then rang the hospital. They were expecting me that morning. Would I be arriving any time soon?

"Well, no. I haven't completed the fasting requirements and, absent that, you wouldn't accept me for the procedure. What about my Tuesday appointment?"

"Nope, there's no Tuesday appointment. No one at the Surgical Admission Suite can help you. Ring the Unit Secretary and hope they can do something."

I rang the Unit Secretary and hoped she could do something. She eventually decided she would make enquiries and I would be rung back.

An hour later the phone rang and Slothful-from-Haematology, the woman suspected by myself as being the cause of all the problems — *You broke it, you fix it!* — told me I was now, miraculously, enrolled for a bone marrow biopsy on the Tuesday.

I asked about the anaesthetic arrangements. Slothful said that she had rung two Doctor Leighs (*I asked how she spelt the name*), without success, but assumed that he would have all arrangements in place for tomorrow.

That was troubling.

Dr. Le was an anaesthetist. Slothful didn't know that.

Dr. Le was a woman. Slothful didn't know that.

Dr. Le's surname was spelled "Le." Slothful didn't know that.

But she wanted me to have full confidence in her arrangements. *I haven't quite got all the facts, but trust me anyway, because I'm a nurse, I'm part of The System, while you're just someone off the street, a temporary blip passing by, and your questions can only be viewed as impertinent. Keep calm and think about something else.*

This was the first time during Stage Two chemotherapy that I'd encountered Big Hospital Attitude, but it wouldn't be the last.

One of the things I'd noticed in the hospital foyer, during my visits to see Dr. Tease, had been the presence of a poster with a photo of a politically correct crowd, hastily rustled up for the purposes of poster-making, and fronted by a smarmy-looking boy who seemed to have no place in the story, unless it was as a *Children Are Our Future* adjunct to this particular campaign. Of course, he might have been the child of Someone Important, or a work experience kid on day release to the photographer, who could only keep him from wandering away by making him the centre of attention in the photo. Whatever.

The poster had been provided by an organisation calling itself "HCSCC," which turned out to be an acronym for "Health and Community Services Complaint Commissioner," a being previously unknown to me.

The substance of the poster was that I had rights when in hospital. I had eight different rights, no less. While these were effectively a government-sponsored "motherhood" statement about things like *Safety* and *Respect*, the last line stood out for me. Number Eight. *Comment*.

I had the right to "comment and / or complain."

Slothful-from-Haematology's cavalier approach to the arrangements for my bone marrow biopsy had left me feeling insecure. And although the poster failed to promise me the right to feel secure, I thought I might mention my concerns to someone in the hierarchy, hopefully someone who cared.

In this modern era of "consumer engagement," one complains — *if one complains at all* — to a Consumer Advisor, a person employed by the hospital to guard its reputation at all costs.

In my experience, this involves them uttering soothing sounds and tut-tutting over undeniably spilt milk, while practicing double-talk and obfuscation in pursuit of the ideal of a sedated and quiescent clientele. The goal is captured in the motto: "KEEP CALM AND THINK ABOUT SOMETHING ELSE."

I narrated my experiences to the Consumer Advisor. She uttered soothing sounds and tut-tutted over the undeniably spilt milk. Then she flicked the problem to the Outpatient Coordinator, who made some enquiries, identified the originating error and — proud as Punch of her quick success — declared the case closed and hung up the phone.

I had just been bounced off the Consumer Advisor wall.

Now, bruised and confused, I tried to take stock. It was Monday. A Tuesday appointment — even if I couldn't be sure of the anaesthetic arrangements — was better than no appointment at all. Rattling the cage at this late stage could unleash a rash of misplaced files and accidentally cancelled appointments. And, lousy as I was feeling, I didn't need the aggravation.

Perhaps I should keep calm and think about something else.

Chapter Four

The bone marrow biopsy went smoothly. The team involved were intrigued to hear the story of how I'd jumped the queue at the last moment. I said it was a long and boring story. They said, "Tell us anyway."

And so, during a few packed minutes, I eked out an expurgated version of events while being folded over, tucked up, pillowed between my knees, injected with a drip, given a tissue so I could cough up a solid without making a mess, rubbed over the target area with antiseptic, draped about the hip, and loaded up with a special cocktail of intravenous drugs. I felt warm and vague, and could only dimly follow the political discussion that dominated the rest of the proceedings.

About a minute later, I was moved to Recovery, where other people were slowly emerging from their pharmacologically-induced fog.

A week later, I met with Dr. Tease, the oncologist, to hear the results.

He peered at his computer screen, quoted a bunch of impressive-sounding numbers, then said, "No doubt about it, you're riddled with leukaemia."

He waited for that to sink in.

I sat, coughed heartily, and waited for him to continue.

"What's happening to you is that the leukaemia is causing swollen lymph nodes, especially in your lungs. The lungs try to rid themselves of the irritation the only way they know how, by coughing. The only way to get rid of the leukaemia and its consequences is... che-mo-therapy."

There was a pause. I listened for a portentous drum roll, but only heard distant giggling from the corridor.

I sat, coughed heartily, and thought: "Chemo-bloody-therapy."

Dr. Tease had been waiting for the right moment and this must have been it. He jumped in with, "You would only have to come in one day a month."

It had been three days a month last time. A two-third reduction was nothing to sniff at.

"On that day, you'd have a combination of a drip and tablets, the other two days you would only take tablets and you could do that at home."

This was the sweetener and it thrilled me, but I played things cautiously. His approach made me think of Kylie, my dental hygienist and a recreational beard fondler. It all started when a patient, a young man with a new beard, invited her to feel it. The softness surprised her and a compulsion was born. The clue with Kylie is that she loves to work the word *hirsute* into a conversation.

Beard fondling can develop into a full-blown mania — *trichotillomania* — which is an obsessive-compulsive disorder, the habit of pulling one's hair out. Kylie denies that she has reached this stage; she's merely engaging in recreational beard fondling, as practised in ancient tribal societies.

Anyway, Kylie's ploy is that, during her treatment of bearded patients, she accidentally spills small amounts of dental treatment substances, such as amalgam, resin or quick-dry cement, on the bristles. The spills are carefully removed and then she finger-combs the beard into a pleasing pattern.

I put up with it all because Kylie is a wonderful dental hygienist and entertaining company. Dr. Tease, on the other hand, not so much.

"I thought I wasn't qualified for the new, improved program."

"I was able to get you a dispensation."

"Thanks."

And here I was saying, Thanks. I'd been taken in by an expert and now I was turning my back on years of protestations that I'd never do this again. I coughed heartily and asked the fatal question, "When do we start?"

Like it was that simple. It wasn't.

First, I needed an exhaustive, personal pharmacopeia, a collection of drugs necessary to offset this side effect, prevent or discourage some other side effect, and inhibit the world of weird, and potentially terminal, physical anomalies associated with chemotherapy.

And so it came to pass that, once I was suitably dosed with prophylactic drugs and potions, and armed with convenient laxatives, such as castor oil and Epsom salts, plus recipes for side orders of chicken soup, barley water, camomile tea, sulphur and molasses, and senega and ammonia, the process began.

My first trip to the chemotherapy ward, back in 2007, had been terrifying. A horseshoe-shaped room was lined with large, electrically-operated armchairs, which were, for the most part, filled with people who did not look well. About half of them wore headgear which suggested their hair had departed.

I took particular notice of this, because I had been told that, during chemo, my hair would fall out and I would lose weight.

That was a trade I was willing to make. My hair had been abandoning the neighbourhood for years anyway. If Detroit had "white flight," I had hair flight. Those that remained received postcards from foreign parts and seemed intent on their own emigration. To lose weight at the price of seeing off the last of them was the bargain of the year.

Of course, neither outcome eventuated, which disappointed my work colleagues, who had tied their sympathy to my hair loss. I was viewed in the office as a chemotherapy failure and possible fraud.

Meanwhile, stainless steel stands were arrayed alongside the armchairs. From these hung plastic bags, linked by plastic tubes to needles in a variety of places: arms, hands, wrists, or shoulders. A range of options were in evidence: clear liquids, red liquids and mysterious black bags.

I was tagged with a plastic band, ushered to an armchair and left sitting nervously for a long time. No one spoke, though eyes flicked around the room as each incumbent tried to calculate how many patients were in worse shape than themselves. It was a small comfort, but I was the healthiest looking person in the room. On the downside, I knew I needn't look for sympathy here.

After a while, a nurse came over, sat at my knee, and read to me from that old medical standard, *Catastrophe and Woe*. It was four pages long and listed just about every disease and calamity of which I had heard, and a good many others.

These were all available as potential side effects to the chemo. By the time she got to the end of page two —which is where it talked about my gonads shrivelling and turning black — I was slumping down in the chair and contemplating more pleasant options: such as the quick and relatively painless death offered when one is mauled by a pack of wild dogs.

I felt awful and they still hadn't done anything to me. But that was about to change.

The nurse ended her reading. There was not, as I expected, a benediction, just the demand that I sign a piece of paper to confirm that *You Have Been Warned*.

"Oh, and here's a copy to take home and share with the neighbours."

Reinforcements arrived in the person of another nurse, who carried a couple of bags of clear liquid, which were hung from a stand. These bags became the focus of intense discussion between the two, as they quoted numbers back and forth.

Then they demanded I tell them my name and date of birth.

Ve haf vays of makink you talk!

I confessed immediately, told them everything: named names, gave up the password, the location of the secret hideout, the radio transmitter, the...

Oh, no, I didn't. That was in a bad dream, one that recurred throughout my first stint at chemo. No matter how much I confessed, it was never enough, and I had to return to the scene of the injections month after month.

A key word that day was "nausea." I was given tablets to take immediately, and more to take at leisure when I couldn't bear the nausea any longer. But I had some trouble with the terminology.

To me, "nausea" was associated with the experiences that marked the end of my school days, when the claim to manhood required heavy drinking. I was quickly acquainted with the toilet facilities of various bars, where I returned their product in a spray aimed in the general direction of an appropriate receptacle. I'd like to point out that there were times when my aim was accurate. Of course, there were other times when the best I could do was clutch a neighbour's front fence as I donated fertiliser for their lawn and garden.

The feelings associated with these events, I called "nausea." Chief among them, and most reliable, was the slow spinning of the room. Also, any churning of the stomach, pressure behind the eyes, or sudden desire to clutch friendly items and hold them close, such as cool ceramic toilet bowls.

I never experienced these feelings while undergoing chemo, and thus didn't make the connection between the tablets I'd been given and the endless talk about "nausea."

Anyway, what sort of nausea is it that can't get up a couple of decent spins of the room?

I did, however, suffer a vague discomfort, a horrible creeping dread, as of having been misplaced within my own body. I don't know how else to describe it, but I felt "wrong." Day and night, I felt misplaced, off balance, out of sorts, just plain wrong.

The few attempts I made to explain this led to strange looks, obvious incomprehension, and a small amount of alarm. When they started edging toward the flaming torches and the pitchforks, I stopped talking about it.

And so it was that I endured the chemotherapy-induced nausea without ever thinking to take the tablets that had been supplied. The feelings were most intense at night. Many times over that six months, I could have been found at three in the morning, closeted in my study, crying.

The other key event of that first day was the various attempts made to insert a needle in one of my veins. These weren't the fine needles used, say, for a blood test. They were closer to the steel tubes used when sedating horses. It was the major skill of chemo ward staff to insert these needles correctly, first time, every time.

The irony of the situation was that many of them — charming, polite, friendly, helpful, knowledgeable, and generous to a fault though they were — lacked that particular skill. For some reason hospital management didn't view this as a disadvantage. However, the patients did and part of the dread that preceded every visit to the chemo ward emerged from our fear of meeting with one of the poorer performers.

My worst experience was the time two nurses required five attempts between them to insert one needle correctly. To my knowledge, the All Hospital record was ten attempts, without success. This probably doesn't sound all that bad, but when you underwent the process daily for three consecutive days, the injury to the obvious target veins accumulated, and the chances of anyone achieving a single, quick, successful piercing diminished steeply.

The discomfort, compounded by the fear that this amateur dart-throwing competition would be a never-ending process, clouded every aspect of life.

By the third month, I was tiring of my role in the pin-cushion Olympics. A particular nurse had latched on to me as a pet project. She was, simultaneously, the most pleasant person and the worst needle jockey of them all. Once she had clocked up three failed attempts and was scouring my arms for a new area in which to drill for oil, I called a halt.

"Stop. No more. Three cracks: that's enough. You've reached the end of your quota. Let's get someone else."

I don't know if she had been waiting for someone to call her out, but she took it in fine style. Her running commentary had included references to her many failures with the large needle as fair cause for reassignment.

Her boss, however, took a different approach. She stepped in as the replacement needle jockey, out of, I suspect, a need to prove her own competence to me, but she came with a steely Big Hospital Attitude. Patients with opinions were unwelcome on her watch and, over the rest of my course of treatment, she let me know at every opportunity.

For my part, I felt that I was a customer, not a pin-cushion. At that time, I'd not heard the phrase "patient-centred care," but in the emotional valley carved out by chemotherapy, I yearned for a little bit of that.

Chapter Five

We arrived at the first month of Stage Two chemotherapy.

The building was familiar, but the staff were almost entirely new. A young nurse settled me in a chair, tagged me with a plastic band, and started the orientation process.

"What do you think we're going to do here today?"

"Inject selected poisons into my system in the hope that they kill all the bad cells and none of the good cells."

My succinct response stopped her flow. She'd had a speech prepared, one which, I'm sure, addressed every aspect of the process, but now she had trouble finding a good starting point. I noticed she was clutching a copy of *Catastrophe and Woe* in one hand.

"I remember that."

"Of course, you've been through all this before."

"Yep."

"Any questions?"

"Nope."

"Well, let's get you started."

The first big difference between Stages One and Two was that the needle used was so much smaller than in olden times. It was a special kind of needle called a "cannula[6]." Once inserted, the sharpened steel part was removed, leaving a tiny, thin, flexible tube inside the vein, which was then taped in place.

And so it began. The nurse plunged the needle into the back of my hand and...

"Oh, no, that's not working. We'll have to try it again."

The second big difference was that this time, when she ran into trouble, the nurse sought immediate assistance from a better qualified needle jockey. During Stage One, she would have gone on ploughing away until she fluked it, or the patient protested, or died in the chair.

Another big change since the Stage One days was the inclusion of amphetamines in my cocktail of tablets during the first three days of the process.

No one explained anything about that to me. I just noticed that on days two and three, in particular, I had enormous energy, way beyond anything I normally experienced. I could put in three hours of hard work in the garden in the time it usually took me to ease myself into that second cup of coffee.

My wife reviewed my private pharmacopeia and worked it out. I understand now how people become addicted to the stuff; it's nice having endless energy, except for the fact you can't sleep. Then, when the tablets ran out, my energy levels dropped through the floor and I wanted to sleep all the time.

---

[6] The word "**cannula**" comes from the Latin, meaning "little reed." Just to make things more interesting for patients, the device can be referred to by either the device name or one of the manufacturers' names. The two I heard used most often were "Jelco" and "Insyte." Doubtless there are others. The standard expression employed by patients was "this thing," as in: "*Can you please take this thing out of my arm?*"

Around my second week, I experienced the onset of constipation. The castor oil and Epsom salts had been slow to kick in.

It was a nasty experience. I became a master of the white-knuckle, gut-clenching, sweat-dripping, low moan recommended as an adjunct to the glacial movement of a piece of jagged granite though the back passage. The process could take up to an hour, not counting the time needed to staunch the haemorrhage afterwards and mop up the blood.

The constipation was a private affair. Not so the flatulence which accompanied it. I started to function as a mobile natural gas producer. The flatus was the worst I'd ever encountered, so thick you could almost see it. The quantity had to be heard to be believed.

It was obvious that the neighbours wanted to complain, but they were afraid to get that close to the house. When I was in the front yard, I could hear them in their homes, praying for a strong breeze.

I once emptied a bus in the City, without trying. You can't open the windows on a modern bus and the people trapped around me all figured there had to be a better way to get home. In the space of two stops an entire busload piled out the doors, gasping for air and muttering angrily about the use of poison gas in the modern era.

Me, I was just grateful for the extra legroom.

I met with Dr. Tease before the start of Month Two. His computer told us that the great bulk of misbehaving white cells had gone. So he planned to increase the dose of chemo drugs.

Fewer problem cells, so even more drugs? Mystified? Yeah, me too. But that's what happened.

It was from about then that the creeping horrors of chemotherapy re-emerged, clouding every waking minute. The effect of the amphetamines faded, as a consequence of habituation, I suppose. There was still a boost on days two and three, but its impact was less every month.

On the other hand, my need for sleep grew exponentially. At one point, I slept (apart from a few short breaks) for forty-eight hours straight. I lost over ten kilos in weight as I was no longer eating. Though greeted with joy, the weight loss proved to be short-lived.

By the end of the fourth month, we knew that the chemo had done a lot of damage. I was now officially anaemic, though I didn't understand the full significance of the fact at the time. The low red cell count left me weak and tired. I could fall asleep at odd times and in odd places.

Then Dr. Tease ordered a course of special injections, one a month for three months. This was some new drug[7] which promised to stimulate my bone marrow activity. A couple of weeks after the initial injection, I had the first of several heavy nose bleeds. These could last for two hours at a time, despite all the pressure and ice packs we brought to bear on the problem.

I got through the fifth month of chemo, but refused to take the third special injection, which I associated with the nose bleeds. Dr. Tease went off on holidays and then the fun really started.

---

[7] **Some new drug**: *Neulasta*, which I've only recently discovered is also known as *Pegfilgrastim*, the significance of which will emerge later in this narrative.

Chapter Six

I had been getting weaker and weaker for months, without having any clear-cut basis for complaint, other than the catch-all of "bloody chemotherapy." Then I got so weak I couldn't walk from the bedroom to the bathroom. I was sleeping up to eighteen hours a day, feeling permanently exhausted. My oncologist was away on holidays, so I was in limbo.

Finally, my desperation became so great I rang the oncologist's assistant and explained the problem. She said to come straight in to the office and they'd take blood tests and work it out from there. Fair enough.

We got a cab to the office. I had to walk about twelve steps, then up a slight ramp to the front door, but I didn't make it. The incline was too much.

I blacked out and smashed, face first, into the ramp. When I came to, I was face down on blood-soaked concrete. Someone was clutching my head, trying to stop the bleeding, while sticking her thumb in my eye.

This occurred in a high traffic area at the back of the hospital. A crowd gathered. A large crowd, including a full range of medical types. Too many cooks is always a bad idea.

I was oblivious to the fact at the time, but I later heard that there was a crowd inside the building watching the crowd outside. A cynic in the group offered odds on who would emerge to take charge of the situation: the higher ranking the medico, the longer the odds. In the end it was an orderly with a British accent and practical common sense. He bellowed and bullied the crowd until he achieved a temporary cohesion of the nerds, sufficient to get me on to a stretcher, then into the Emergency Department.

That was the first time I found myself indebted to the "menial" staff of a large hospital. It wouldn't be the last.

A doctor stitched up my head, in a rough and cheerful fashion. My wife, who spent many years working with plastic surgeons, said any one of them would have put twenty stitches in a wound that size. This guy only had time for seven. Still, I'm not complaining; he was a nice guy.

The blood test results arrived. Normal levels for haemoglobin in adult males is 130 to 170. I had 39, which explained a lot of things.

This reading set off two streams of activity: one, transfusions to increase my haemoglobin levels; the other, a search to uncover the reason for the loss of blood.

Have you had any nose bleeds lately?

"Yep, heaps of them, some lasting for hours."

Make a note: If a nose bleed lasts more than twenty minutes, get yourself into Emergency so they can cauterize the wound. Apparently, people die from nose bleeds.

This short exchange led to a junior Ear Nose and Throat surgeon getting involved and shoving lots of stainless steel up my nose. After all the stretching, I can now fit my mobile phone inside my left nostril, which is handy.

Have you been shitting black?

Yep, for about a month.

It turns out that black turds are caused by half-digested blood. This is considered a bad thing, so tell your doctor.

I was instructed that, following my next dump, I should run out and get a nurse to come look at the proceeds. This occurred about 4:30am a couple of days later and the Chinese night shift nurse had the privilege of examining my droppings and writing a detailed description in my notes.

About the time that the conversation in the Emergency area turned to black turds, the doctor had finally managed to get a line into a vein and started with the first transfusion. This had been a difficult and painful process because, when you haven't a lot of blood, you don't have much in the way of veins to target. There were only a few false starts, but the shock was wearing off and I had begun to feel emotional.

Meanwhile, Dr. Dreadful, a plump haematologist-in-training, acting on some half-remembered lecture of years ago, decided to contribute her own procedure. She whipped on a blue rubber glove, snapped it at the wrist in an authoritative manner, shoved and prodded me into rolling on my side, then slammed her small (but perfectly formed) fist up my arse.

Most of the air left my lungs in a strangled cry, my eyes bulged and I started whimpering softly. I had a vision of myself, in a white dress, riding a horse along an unspoilt beach. In the distance a cathedral bell tolled and I could hear an angelic choir warming up the *Hallelujah Chorus*.

To make things clear, I had been a bum virgin for five days short of sixty-two years; this despite twelve years of Catholic education, eight years with the Marist Brothers[8], two years as an altar boy[9], three years as a Boy Scout, offers from men who picked me up when hitchhiking, and something similar repeated by GPs over the years.

---

[8] The 2017 *Royal Commission into Institutional Responses to Child Sexual Abuse* reported that over 20% of all Marist Brothers since 1950 had been accused of child sexual abuse and that the order had paid out over $31million in compensation since 1980.

[9] The Catholic authorities admitted to the Royal Commission that there had been thousands of claims of abuse against their officials and that they had paid out over $268million in compensation since 1980.

I always declined, modestly, and suggested that I was happy to wait until I was sent to prison. Anyone who spent time in their youth dodging paedophiles will understand my view. I had been a bum virgin for almost sixty-two years and now I was... buggered.

The other achievement of Dr. Dreadful was that by forcing me on to my side, she dislodged the cannula in my arm. In a room full of medical people, I was the only one to notice. They probably expect to see their patients crying.

When I finally recovered my voice, and was able to ask if the drip was working, they leapt at the chance to offer an expert opinion. Crowded voices rose to a crescendo of agreement that, no, there seemed to be a problem.

No one asked how the problem had arisen, and I was left to recline, like a lone cut flower in an autumn garden bed, and enjoy the moment, as the doctor probed, with a piece of sharpened steel, for another working vein.

The black turd blood must be coming from somewhere. How about an endoscopy?

This took place a couple of days later. It was an interesting event. They took a small fire hose, with periscope and torpedo tubes attached, and blasted their way through the soft tissue at the back of my throat, all the way down to my balls. The report I overheard later was that nothing out of the ordinary had been found.

The endoscopy failed to explain the reason for the black turds. The suggestion that the blood was somehow connected to the nose bleeds didn't ring true for me, as the pattern and duration of the one didn't match the other.

They continued to pump blood into me. Two or three units a day. Toward the end, they were slamming it in at a rate of one every two hours. Early on, they were more cautious and I slowly grew accustomed to being tethered to a drip most of the time.

By my final day in hospital, I was feeling chipper; the best I'd felt in months. My chipperness was offset by boredom, however, so I improvised some street theatre.

My wife had delivered some things from home in a cute little pink and white bag. I spent hours, standing at the door to my room, with only my belly protruding into the corridor, the little bag held out of sight, waiting until a passer-by, usually a visitor, came along.

Once I achieved eye contact, I would whip out the bag and ask, "Does this bag suit me?"

Some people laughed, but most adopted the side-stepping shuffle-with-panicked-gaze, reminiscent of many visitors I saw at the psych hospital where I worked in the 1970s.

My major concern on being discharged from the hospital later that day was: Where will I find shoes to match my bag?

Chapter Seven

At the time of my discharge, all seemed well. I was placed on a follow-up regime of twice-weekly blood tests in order to monitor the state of my haemoglobin. A week later, it was 99.

Four days after that, I had another blood test. The haemoglobin level was down to 77. That's a drop of 22 in three days, with no cuts, nose bleeds or other event to account for it. At that rate, I could reasonably expect to be back on the blood-soaked concrete within the week.

This led to a transfusion, then another blood test two days later. At that point, I was back to feeling dreadful.

I had the blood test early in the afternoon, then waited for a phone call. I sat in the entrance to the hospital, ate three quarters of a salad roll, and observed the passing parade.

About 3:30pm, someone from The Blood Book[10] (a mysterious person who monitors potentially problematic test results) rang, told me my haemoglobin was 62, and that I should admit myself to the Emergency Department.

I had to ask how one did that. The assumption that I should know proved to be a hallmark of many experienced hospital people: *I know, therefore everyone knows. What's wrong with you?*

By following the instructions given, I arrived at a heavily fortified window with the word TRIAGE above it. I was instructed to wait while the young lady behind the fortifications took a phone call.

---

[10] More about this later.

I stood as long as I could, but, fearing another collapse, moved to a seat in the adjacent waiting area. This provoked outrage from behind the armoured glass. There was paperwork to be completed and I was failing to adhere to The System.

I explained that I would rather sit down than fall down, which provoked a barrage of medical advice from an interesting assemblage of persons in the waiting area: truly, a surreal moment.

Though I didn't recognise it at the time, I was being introduced to two important facts. 1) I had ceased to be a victim, a patient, or a person-in-need, and was now a slab of meat whose purpose in life was to obey the officers of The System. And 2), I had entered a world governed by The Rules. I was to be confronted more fully by these facts later when I landed in Ward 6B.

A cheerful man arrived with a trolley, hoisted me aboard, and we set sail for the crowded marketplace of the Emergency Department, where, over a space of some three hours I met about thirty people, answered several hundred questions, received a unit of blood, engaged in repartee with Tony-the-Gastroenterologist and Luke-the-Haematologist, and was fingered up the arse several times.

In the midst of all this, a young woman carrying a foot-long splinter of wood, with a swab attached, arrived. She demanded a turn at testing my reaction to having things shoved up my arse. By the time I was removed from the Emergency Department, I felt I had just completed a long season in prison.

The consensus of the Tony and Luke discussions was that I was not losing blood internally, that the black turds I had been producing for weeks were not in fact black, and that chemotherapy had destroyed my body's ability to reproduce red blood cells at the required pace.

Luke made it clear that blood is a precious resource and not to be wasted on people with haemoglobin above 80 or thereabouts. The Law of Diminishing Returns applies and I could expect limited support in the future.

Given that I needed a minimum haemoglobin level of 100 to function safely, this news came as a shock[11].

From there, I was promoted to Ward 6B. The fact that nursing staff standing nearby all averted their eyes at the mention of my destination should have served as a warning, but I was busy thinking about haemoglobin and the Law of Diminishing Returns.

My portion of Ward 6B was in a corner, adjacent a window with a pleasing view of a brick wall. When I arrived, there were many people present. I struggled to work out which were patients, and which were relatives, neighbours, salesmen, or parole officers. The security guards wear a distinctive uniform, which helped. The growl of the televisions blended nicely with the roar of conversation, some of which took place in English.

There was a bed, but no chair. There was a yellow concertinaed curtain which could screen me from the rest of Eastern Europe. I promptly closed it. This led to a delightful game where nurses would open the curtain and I would close it again. Homer Simpson would have felt comfortable here.

My wife dropped by with a few things, including a couple of small chocolate bars, standard security items for diabetics.

---

[11] The **Rule of 80** became a nightmare for me in the days that followed. Put simply, the idea is that, if a patient with functioning bone marrow has a haemoglobin base of 80, the normal work of their bone marrow in producing additional red cells will lift them back to their version of normal. The second part of the Rule 80, largely unknown to interns in Adelaide, is that, if the patient has no (repeat *no*) functiong bone marrow, the base of 80 quickly becomes 70, then 60, then 39 and you collapse in the street. Thinking of England, whistling Dixie, or holding your mouth a certain way doesn't help. Oh, and good luck in explaining that to an intern afflicted with a personal sense of omniscience.

I was given a second unit of blood. By the time that was done, the crowd had thinned, though chatter continued until about midnight. From there, we were down to the flicker of television screens reflecting off the shiny floor, and the repeated demands of a European gentleman who had a strong interest in "the syrup." I took this to be some form of painkiller.

The nurses didn't share his view of how much he needed and a battle of wills played out over the rest of the night. I heard one nurse forcefully explain that there was a button he could press to gain her attention. Whether or not he pressed the button I don't know, but if so he supplemented it with sustained *wooh-wooh-wooh* groans. It was an interesting vocal pattern.

I couldn't sleep. I couldn't sit in a chair, as these are reserved (I think) for patients who have visits from parole officers. I sat on the side of the bed and dangled my legs, my feet half a metre off the ground, and tried to discern the source of the various noises.

For several hours I sat, entranced, swinging my legs back and forth in an irresponsible fashion, while deciding that this noise was air-conditioning, but that noise was electronic hum from a television set.

It was an exciting time, interrupted only by nursing visits for obs[12] and further demands for "the syrup."

About 5:30am I recognised that I was slipping into a state of hypoglycaemia[13]. A quick test showed a reading of 3.7, which was

---

[12] **Obs**: The standard abbreviation for the routine observations taken of patients: blood pressure, temperature, pulse.

[13] Every cell in our bodies burns **glucose** as a fuel. Most people need to maintain between 4.1 and 6.0mmol/L (that's millimoles per litre) in their blood to function effectively. [In some other countries they measure it in mg/dL (milligrams per decilitre).] If your blood glucose level (BGL) drops below 4.0, you have entered a state of hypoglycaemia, or a "hypo". It is important to treat a hypo quickly to stop the BGL from falling even lower and the person becoming seriously unwell.

to be expected, given I had eaten only the final quarter of my lunchtime salad roll since being admitted to hospital some fourteen hours earlier.

I ate a small Turkish Delight, then sucked on a cough lolly for good measure. Not an approach recommended by endocrinologists, I know, but there was no alternative.

That's when I started to think about home. If I was home, I could get some real food. If I was home, I could sit in a chair. If I was home, I could get some sleep in a comfortable bed. If I was home, I wouldn't have to hear about "the syrup." Despite the many attractions of Ward 6B, this idea, of being at home, was growing on me.

About 7:30am, someone delivered a tray. I was sat, looking at it, having just identified one paper bag as containing a slice of cold toast, which might serve to help me take my morning tablets, when a Bright Young nurse appeared.

She'd just learned that I was a diabetic who managed his own insulin, which fact startled her. Slabs of meat don't "manage" anything, least of all insulin, not in Ward 6B. She was here to take a blood glucose reading of her own, in accordance with The Rules.

I asked her what my blood glucose reading had been at 5:30am. This question created momentary panic, as it came from somewhere outside the script she had been following. I let her down gently and told her the numbers, which triggered a second panic state. To her credit, she recognised that this was in the realm of hypoglycaemia, but that was a condition above her pay grade. She fled.

Shortly after, a higher-ranking Overbearing nurse arrived to straighten me out. I would not be administering any insulin to myself until a doctor had reviewed my dosage, she announced. In her understanding, the sole possible cause of hypoglycaemia is a patient taking an incorrect dose of insulin. And she had ways of fixing that, never you mind.

I bit my tongue, hard, then suggested that there might be an alternative explanation... such as the fact that I'd had close to nothing to eat in fourteen hours.

Overbearing's first reaction was to declare me a liar. She described an imaginary meal I must have eaten at 6:00 the night before. I informed her that I had been locked in combat with the Hopoate[14] Attack Battalion in the Emergency Department at that time. The rugby reference might have been lost on her, but the mention of Emergency was enough to make her wonder what time I had arrived at Ward 6B.

She went off to investigate and soon returned, in a state of outrage that I had not been given a meal. The important thing now, in keeping with The Rules, was the institution of a witch-hunt to find a scapegoat. There was no apology.

Me, I just wanted to eat the cold toast.

Overbearing departed, but was quickly replaced by Bright Young. Despite the fact she knew I was a diabetic, one who had recently slipped into hypoglycaemia, despite the fact I had a slice of toast, recently coated with cheap marmalade, in my hand and inches from my mouth, she demanded that I submit to a full set of obs. Now. In accordance with The Rules.

I put the toast down and submitted to the process, despite a growing irritation with the level of stupidity on display in Ward 6B. It was about then that I decided to go home.

---

[14] I was emboldened to leave this reference to John Hopoate in the book after watching the 2004 movie *The Last Shot*, in which Tony Shalhoub plays a mobster related to John Gotti. He exclaims how he hates poor sportsmanship while watching a video of the incident in which Hopoate thrust his finger into a guy's anus during a 2001 rugby match.

I rang my wife and warned her. She arrived with clothes and I got dressed. I still had a cannula in the back of my hand. My wife found someone to inform that we were leaving and requested assistance with the cannula.

Bright Young and Overbearing shuffled into the background, and a Large Bully nurse arrived to snap at me about The Rules and how a mere slab of meat couldn't make a decision, any decision, without the assistance of an officer of The System, and that I would sit right there until a small phalanx of more senior people had taken turns at rejecting my outrageous request.

I asked Large Bully for assistance in removing the cannula. She refused. It was obvious that her tactic was Bluff and Bluster. She intended to stonewall me, wear me down, and eventually impose her will on me.

I pulled out the cannula.

That was an interesting moment. Blood spurted, fountain-like, from the back of my hand. We went through a box of tissues in stemming the flow, without any gesture of help from Large Bully. Blood seeped from the tissues, down my fingers and into big splashes on the floor.

I was still sitting uncomfortably on the side of the bed, feet dangling above the blood spray, when I noticed that the adjacent bed was unoccupied and made up. It was a low bed, a place where I could sit, touch the floor with my feet, and briefly feel like a normal person. I moved to that bed.

This caused heightened outrage. How dare I sit comfortably, while bleeding all over the place. No concern was shown by Large Bully, not for me, but she had deep concerns about another patient, whose arrival was expected shortly. She demanded again that I get off that bed. I told her I wanted a chair, and one was located within seconds, despite the absence of my parole officer.

I had just moved to this chair, when Dr. Dreadful arrived. I hoped she would model the calming, thoughtful behaviour of an aspiring specialist. Instead we got a louder version of Large Bully. Aggressive, belligerent, angry. All bully and no brains.

A real doctor arrived later and managed a calm and reasonable tone, which was a pleasant change. She had a consultant in tow, who asked three or four inane questions, which helped illustrate the pointlessness of the process.

My wife was having her say when Dr. Dreadful snapped that it was impossible for me to leave Ward 6B.

Really?

I stood up, collected my bag, and left.

In the midst of her tirade, Dr. Dreadful had announced that, by walking out of the hospital, I would be breaking the nexus between my past relationship with Dr. Tease and any future problems I might have. In short, it would be into the outer darkness for me, in which place I could expect wailing and gnashing of teeth.

I had trouble believing her threats, but you never know.

When my wife emerged from the hospital, she was clutching some blood test forms. These reflected the twice-weekly arrangement that existed before I broke the nexus. I had no idea where I now stood with my oncologist, but decided to show up for a blood test the next day in order to find out.

I wrote an e-mail to Dr. Tease to explain how things had unfolded, from my point of view. (I had no doubt he would be hearing another version of the story from people who needed to cover themselves.) The next morning, I fronted up for a blood test and was relieved to find myself treated me in a kindly fashion. The e-mail I'd written had been passed around. There was some embarrassment over how I'd been treated, but no surprise.

Chapter Eight

Another week, another blood test. This one showed a haemoglobin of 71. So I went in on a Good Friday for a blood transfusion. It was strange to find myself in a tiny pocket of activity within a darkened building. The staff were light-hearted and cheerful: maybe something to do with the chocolate Easter eggs they were consuming.

The next day I felt flat. The day after that — Easter Sunday — there would be no uprising[15]. On the contrary, I felt dangerously weak, and predicted that my haemoglobin level was in the low sixties.

We took a taxi to the hospital, for my third admission in less than two months. I slumped in a plastic chair while my wife translated my situation into nursing-ese for the benefit of Triage.

A young woman arrived with a bed, which she slapped into shape with a series of clicks and clacks, before ordering me aboard. I rolled onto my back, like a tired puppy ready for one last tummy-tickle before bed.

The usual Emergency Department groups gathered to peer and prod at me. A doctor ordered a blood test, and a saline drip to boost my blood pressure, which was then down to 80.

The blood test result showed my haemoglobin as a robust 63. Dr. Good decided that the two units of blood per visit, which I had been given previously, were inadequate, and ordered three units of blood at a rate of one every three hours. Which meant I wouldn't get home on Sunday.

---

[15] This event took place on the centenary of the **1916 Easter Uprising** in Ireland. I couldn't resist the little play on words.

Once the first unit of blood was plugged into my arm, I was moved to Ward 6A, Room 1, which is at the far end, away from most people, they said, so that my sobbing wouldn't disturb them, they said. Or it might have been "snoring." I'm not sure which.

I was still settling in when I was informed that Dr. Good had decided to add a litre of saline over twelve hours on account of my poor creatinine[16] levels. That moved things out to fifteen hours, assuming a fairly swift changeover between units. Ha ha ha.

Each changeover took at least an hour, which puzzled me at first. Then I noticed that the nurse who eagerly volunteered to collect the blood, one unit at a time, was a smoker. Seems she was enjoying an extended smoke break under the cover of performing an act of kindness.

The Ward hummed along. Evening approached, which meant time for meds and insulin. Which meant a battle looming.

Smoker Nurse required that I hand control of my meds and insulin to her, immediately, in accordance with The Rules. She had the regretful tone of a young mother who, on taking a sharp knife away from a child, says, "I know you're having fun, but this is too dangerous for you to play with."

I politely refused her request, explaining that I had managed my meds and insulin, seven days a week, for a decade, and felt most comfortable continuing with what I knew.

She persisted. "It's a Rule of this ward that all meds and insulin are controlled by nursing staff."

Ah, ward-centred nursing. So much for Person-Centred Care, with or without the caps.

---

[16] **Creatinine** is a waste product that comes from the normal wear and tear on muscles of the body.

"Sorry. That's not going to happen."

She sighed, then graciously explaining the situation, as one would to an especially simple patient, said, "We had a woman in here last year who insisted on handling her own insulin. We let her. Then she injected a full dose of fast-acting insulin, instead of the usual 24-hour slow-release version. Ever since then we've had this Rule."

So, one foolish mistake (or was it deliberate?) by one person and the rest of humankind were to be bound forever by the iron law of the Medes and the Persians.

"I'll feel more comfortable looking after it myself, but thanks anyway."

She departed, leaving me to contemplate my sins, alone. Five minutes later, she was back. She'd rung Dr. Dreadful, who'd said something to the effect of, Let him do what he likes, just write it up as "Self Administered". The tone of the message, as delivered to me, was: "Let him kill himself and we'll have one less idiot to worry about."

I leapt to my feet and applauded. Hallelujah! Peace and common sense reigned. It was Easter Sunday after all.

But that wasn't the end of it. Smoker Nurse now started a childish game of *Gotcha!* with every round of observations. She added a blood glucose reading to the roster and, after checking each reading, demanded that I tell her the number. If I was wrong, to her mind, it would prove... something. I don't know what. However, I got it right, plus or minus a maximum of two, every time.

My favourite round of *Gotcha!* came less than an hour after I'd eaten a meal. I considered the blood test an exercise in absurdity, but bit my tongue.

"What's the reading?" she asked.

"Double figures," was my reply.

"Eleven point one."

That soon after eating, it had to be in double figures. The recommended time lapse before testing is two hours.

I asked her, "What did you learn from that test?"

She had no answer.

Perhaps ungraciously, I added, "I wouldn't have bothered."

Smoker Nurse stalked from the room and, with a parting snort, said, "That's because you're glycaemically irresponsible."

I later looked up the term on Google and drew exactly zero hits for the expression. This adversarial version of patient centred care gave hospital staff another impressive weapon with which they could score points over patients: *glycaemic irresponsiblity*.

And I was to be the poster child for the condition.

I'm still wondering if there'll be royalties.

The night was long and tedious. Hourly "obs" by a nurse from Sierra Leone provided me with something to read up about on my phone. I felt like a dog, chained to the fence by the drip in my arm. When marking time late at night, I like to pace up and down, but three steps didn't do it for me.

I must have fallen asleep about five o'clock. I was woken at six by someone wanting to take blood. I told her I'd only just gotten the blood and was hoping to do a couple more laps with it before they took it back. She was a traditional no-nonsense nurse and had a needle in a vein, blood in a tube, and was gone again in a flash. I went back to sleep.

I was woken about seven by a repeated shriek from the infusion pump. This electrical device-on-a-stand controlled the rate at which fluid was fed into my arm. The shrieking started if I bent my arm, creating a kink in the line. Standing with my arm hanging straight down usually cured the condition.

Not this time. The shrieking machine ground on and on. It was a loud noise which I couldn't escape, as I was tethered to the source. On and on it screamed. I practised swearing. I practised swearing LOUDLY. No joy.

The noise was creating a problem for me; I feared bleeding from the ears. In desperation, I fingered my hair into a cockscomb, pulled the plug out of the wall, then, with my hair on end and the arse out the back of my frock, I hobbled along the corridor, pushing the shrieking Dalek in front of me.

My wife later asked why I didn't have my jocks on. I told her that hospital beds all slope toward the feet. As I slid down, my jocks would ride up. They would take my gronicles in a stranglehold, and squeeze until the colour drained from my face and all the joy from my life.

It was quiet in the corridor. My shuffling progress functioned as a travelling fire alarm, arousing irritation in an overworked nurse. She rushed over and massaged various parts of the Dalek until it fell silent.

I was ever so grateful and said so. She indicated she'd prefer my absence to my gratitude. Suitably chastened, I returned to my room and plugged the Dalek into the wall. It took instant offence and began shrieking again.

This time I didn't delay, but pulled the plug out and shuffled into the corridor.

Irritated Nurse put in a prompt appearance, glanced at the screen on the Dalek, and shouted at me that it wanted to be plugged into the wall. I told her that that was what had set it off the last time. She didn't have the patience for conversation, but turned me around and pushed me toward my room.

This brought my exact state of dress to her attention. She now combined irritation over my idiocy with irritation over my naked arse, and pushed me forward while attempting a complicated double fold at the back of my frock.

Once in my room, Irritated Nurse slammed the plug into the wall and started to unfold a gesture of triumph, except the Dalek continued to shriek.

I didn't say anything.

She massaged various parts of the Dalek.

I didn't say anything.

Eventually the Dalek fell silent.

I couldn't say anything nice, so I didn't say anything at all. My mother would have been proud of me.

Chapter Nine

The morning shift arrived in the person of an anxious young woman. She was a replacement for an absentee and wanting to do well. I had an impression of an over-eager puppy, or a mechanical clockwork toy — wind it up, point it in the right direction, and it would run all day.

The problem arose from the concept of "right direction." To Clockwork Puppy that meant The Rules. And The Rules said she would have total control of my meds and insulin.

Ahh, not again...

Explaining didn't help. Pointing her to The Book and the lessons to be drawn from yesterday's practice didn't help. Clockwork Puppy had a limited capacity for thinking outside the box. Eventually I achieved a stalemate, which prompted her to go in search of a higher authority.

An older, larger, wiser nurse appeared; she played an excellent Good Cop. She sat alongside me, instead of opposite, in the traditional adversarial position. She opened by distancing herself from the problem, explaining that she understood but Clockwork Puppy was rigid, bound by The Rules. She looked for common ground, settling on football allegiances and related interests. She laughed at my jokes. She became my friend. She offered a compromise — I could handle the meds and insulin, while a nurse observed. Then she appealed for my indulgence in settling Clockwork Puppy's insecurities.

It was straight out of the textbook chapter, *When Dealing with an Awkward Old Bastard*.

I agreed to the compromise, with Clockwork Puppy to be the witness.

About a minute later, Clockwork Puppy burst into the room, ostensibly to observe the administration of the insulin, but mostly to mark her triumph in the battle for control.

Oh, and she had two tablets for me. These had come from the hospital pharmacy.

She announced them by their pharmaceutical names, an exercise lost on me. My G.P. always referred to them by their trade name. The prescription always stated the trade name. The pharmacist spoke of them by their trade name. I had a rigid trade name orientation, as do the bulk of the population, a fact which most of the staff at this hospital appeared to be unaware.

I had already explained to Clockwork Puppy, several times, that I had all the pills I needed stored in a seven-day Pill Dispenser in my bag. I would take my morning tablets, with my breakfast, as I had done, seven days a week, lo these many years.

Perhaps she was deaf. Perhaps she wasn't listening. Perhaps the lift never reached the top floor. I don't know, but she insisted on handing me two tablets and proclaiming that they made up a small part of my morning medication; the rest would turn up later.

I didn't try to explain the dangers of dispensing medication piecemeal. The morning tablets — *all* the morning tablets — were meant to be taken at the same time, as they had been for a decade.

Once again I'd run into Big Hospital Attitude. She was a nurse: she was here to tell me things; she was not here to listen to me.

I made another attempt and explained that I took my insulin at 8:30am and 8:30pm.

Clockwork Puppy announced that she would return at 8:30am, then bounced out of the room.

I dropped the two tablets down the sink.

And that was it, the show was over. Clockwork Puppy got caught up in the tribulations of another patient in the next room and the question of my insulin — apparently, for her, a life-and-death matter just minutes earlier — was now forgotten.

Come 8:30am and I was on my own, administering my insulin to myself, as I had done for many years; on time, correct dose, correct insulin type; no fuss, no bother. Had I waited for Clockwork Puppy to provide the dose I needed, I would be waiting still. And for me, that really is a matter of life-and-death.

Breakfast came and went. A slice of cold toast topped with cheap marmalade. It had such a familiar look to it that I grew nostalgic. I took my tablets, chewed on the rubbery toast, and thought of better times.

By now I had completed the transfusions and was drip-free, seated on the side of the bed, feet resting on the overway base, facing the door to the room, in a state of reverie. Or contemplation. Or meditation. Or wool-gathering, as my wife would have it. I looked up and Dr. Dreadful, suddenly framed in the doorway, loomed into view, a dark harbinger of disaster.

I cacked myself on the spot.

Something about my demeanour provoked her to introduce herself again. I nodded politely. She said that my haemoglobin level was 74, a clear advance on 63, but not quite what we'd hoped for from three units of blood. Her supervisor, Dr. Good, had decided to administer another three units at a rate of one every three hours.

If, at the end, my haemoglobin was above 80, I could go home.

I maintained an agreeable grimace, all the time nodding and praying she'd leave before discovering what condition my condition was in. I feared my disgrace being exposed to crowds of hospital workers and becoming the substance of daily conversation. *Never seen the like in all my born days: he seemed like such a nice man an' all. You can never really tell...*

Dr. Dreadful left. I bolted to deposit a large turd in the toilet. After my best efforts at cleaning up, I was left with a stained bed sheet. A friendly young nurse agreed to replace it with a fresh supply, while I hid in the shower.

The remainder of the day unravelled slowly. Three units at three hours each, with intervals between — never more than an hour and a half at a time — stretched out the day for me. I had hopes of going home that evening, but it wasn't to be. The original idea of taking a blood test three hours after the last transfusion had been completed was abandoned. That could wait for tomorrow.

I drew the curtain, closed the door, shut the blinds, and retreated to bed. My sleep patterns had remained disrupted ever since the excitement of Ward 6B, but exhaustion took over and I experienced an approximation of a good night's sleep, the occasional obs notwithstanding.

I was awake at 5:00am and perched on the side of the bed, ready for my blood test. I maintained this state for the next three and half hours, until someone finally wandered in to take my blood. Then I had to wait for the results.

At 11:30am Dr. Good arrived. He said my haemoglobin was 100 and that I could go home. My joy was unconfined. I called for dancing in the streets. I bestowed Dr. Good with blessings, immediate promotion, a medal, or at least a Gold Star. He seemed happy with that.

It was Tuesday and my Easter was finally over.

Chapter Ten

I developed a persistent sore on my lower lip. I thought it was a cold sore and treated it with a cream which came with the promise of a cure, or at least some relief. For a while the sore responded well, shrinking and no longer bleeding. Then it flared up again. More cream, some improvement, then another flare up.

This went on for weeks, until I took the problem to my General Practitioner. He referred me to a dermatologist, a strange man with furtive habits which made me nervous.

In my experience, most doctors type into a computer, or if technologically challenged, scribble notes in spidery doctor scrawl onto a piece of paper. Dr. Strange spent most of the consultation clutching a small Dictaphone into which he would speak part of a sentence, hit Rewind, play back those few words, speak a few more, hit Rewind, play back the few extra words, and so on. He recorded copious, detailed notes which had me squirming in my seat.

Eventually he got to the point: I had a cancerous growth on my lower lip. It had to go, but he didn't want the job of taking it out, and referred me instead to another dermatologist.

This one was young, female, bright and cheerful. She told me that the cancer would not go away by itself. It had to be removed, forcibly. She could do the job with a sharp knife, or she could utilise her shiny new laser machine. My problem was a perfect opportunity for her to demonstrate the power of her toy. One short treatment and I would be free of the problem for ever.

I could only say *Yes, Please*, and accept the booking offered.

A few days later I found myself in a room with Dr. Laser, an older nurse and the shiny new machine. The setup was reminiscent of the CT scanner, except there was no sci-fi hum from the machine or vacuum-hiss from the doors.

I was hoisted aboard the tray, laid flat on my back, had my head fixed in position with a couple of heavy coach bolts, my chin strapped to prevent movement, and told to relax.

Over the course of many treatments, I've become almost blasé about surgical processes. I like to think of myself as being cool, but it's really just fatalism. If they're going to kill me here, well, there's nothing much I can do about it. I might as well take a deep breath and relax.

So, I took a deep breath and I relaxed.

I'm sure you've heard how laser surgery is clean, precise, quick, effective, and pain free. Yep, it's all that. What they don't tell you is that it can be really disgusting.

In this case, the goal was to slice a couple of layers of tissue from my lower lip. Simple, right? No, not really.

The official claim is that laser beams can vaporise any soft tissue which has a high water content: a lower lip, for example. What really happens is that layers of lip are burned off slowly, one at a time, like a wildly overcooked steak on a backyard barbecue.

Picture, if you will, a steak tossed onto a hot plate and left until it is black and smoking. I mean charred all the way through, with no residual juices; carbon in the form of small black lumps; charcoaled flesh.

This is what happened to me. One layer of lip was charred, then the process stopped while the ash was scraped from the wound. Then another blast, another scraping, and on we went.

Barbecued lip, everyone's favourite.

The older nurse clutched my hand and told me how well I was doing, even though I wasn't doing anything, a fact which fed into a growing sense of paranoia.

Dr. Laser was chatty, cheerful, enthusiastic about progress; even the scraping of the ashes seemed to be a source of joy for her.

Had I been able to speak without fear of being sliced through the mouth by stray laser beams, I might have joined in, but as things were I remained frozen in fixed grimace.

I had a fleeting childhood memory: my mother threatening that, if the wind changed direction, I would be left with that face as a permanent expression.

I could only breathe through my nose, which is positioned alarmingly close to my lip, from whence arose a stream of smoke. I could but inhale my own flesh as it emerged from the deathbed of a layer of lip, and drifted into the atmosphere like the evidence of a group of naughty schoolboys huddled behind the toilets with a packet of cigarettes.

I was, unexpectedly, practicing a form of cannibalistic inhalation, with my charred and smouldering lip an offering at the altar of modern medical science.

Clean? Precise? Quick? Not so much. The lip scraping was the slowest part. I assume Dr. Laser was being careful not to rip up large slabs of tissue by accident and for that I'm grateful.

The one constant was the bleeding. A slow ooze of blood from the scraped lip began during the surgery and continued unabated for some nineteen days. Yeah, nineteen, I counted them. That was nineteen days where I coated the lip with an ointment to cover and protect the open wound. Nineteen days that I was off work. And although I'd sent emails describing the drama, the evidence before the eyes of my co-workers when I finally made it back to the office was of a clean, healed lower lip.

Photos. I should have taken photos, right at the start, a lesson I was slow to learn. I'd failed to manage the understanding of my workmates, especially my boss, and my veracity began to be doubted.

Chapter Eleven

From lips to eyes. I noticed my eyesight was less sharp than it had once been, so I made an appointment to be assessed for new glasses.

The process began in a darkened backroom where a young woman seated me in front of something I'd never seen before, a large bubble, like a huge boiled egg, with a tiny eye hole located near the top of the outer circumference.

It was soon obvious that she had a limited grasp of how to use this machine. Instead of lowering it to a height comfortable for the customer, she kept shoving my head from behind, in an attempt to have the mountain come to Mohammed.

Then my mobile phone rang. It was another woman from the same optometrist's office. This one wanted me to know that we had an appointment and where exactly was I?

I found it difficult to provide a precise geographical location, but eventually convinced her that I was somewhere in the building. She decided that this was sufficient and agreed to leave me to my fate.

Shoving Woman persisted with her idiotic technique. I had to ask her three times — no, that's *three* times — before she finally desisted from her shove-head-*Bang*!-into-the-machine routine.

I located the controls at the base of the egg and worked out how to lower the eye hole to a comfortable height. Some pictures were obtained.

Shoving Woman complained about the quality of the pictures. Later the optometrist would complain about the quality of the pictures. I have had limited experience with Soviet Surplus machines, but suspect that my fear of further shove-head-*Bang!*-into-the-machine events contributed to a high level of anxiety and a corresponding tension about the target area of my eyes. This might have affected the quality of the pictures.

From here I was led, blinking, into the light of the optometrist's office, where I was seated safely against a wall. The optometrist engaged in small talk, mostly focussed on the time elapsed since my last visit to this establishment.

I attempted to explain the trauma of Stage One and the shove-head-*Bang!*-into-the-machine routine, but there was money to be collected and he was eager to move on. He waved off my comments and swung into action.

Huge metal-framed goggles pivoted on a hinge and landed somewhere around the latitude of my eyes. A curved plastic-coated baffle, affixed to the leading edge, clamped itself to my skull. I suspect that other people, people with more hair, people with a traditional fringe, say, found this baffle a comfort as it protected them from the impact of the weighty goggles, but as the baffle locked on, limpet-like, to my bare skull, I found myself a prisoner.

There was no give. When the optometrist attempted to slide the device sideways — to obtain a more convenient location — a first layer of skin lifted and threatened to peel from my face. I wrenched myself away and repositioned closer to the place I guessed he wanted me to be.

This became a cycle, as he repeated the face-sliding, skin-peeling approach, while I countered with head-wrenching-and-repositioning. Eventually I must have guessed correctly (or maybe he just tired of the head-wrenching-and-repositioning), and we entered upon a long session of *Which-is-better-one-or-two?*

Then I was ejected and returned to the impressive frame collection area, where we went through the *Pick-a-frame* routine and the *Paint-a-black-dot-on-the-glasses* routine and the *You-can-pay-a-deposit-now* routine. I was told I would receive a text on my phone when the glasses were ready.

In due course the text arrived and I presented myself at the front desk. A pair of glasses were handed to me. I tried them on. Long vision was excellent. Close reading vision was appalling. I had double vision.

The young woman went through an impressive performance, designed to convince me that the glasses were fine, but there was something weird about how I positioned them on my face. Black dots were drawn and rubbed out. The lenses were aligned against a ruler, several times. The glasses were fed into a machine. There was much measuring and weighing and sighing and repositioning and re-angling until I cracked under the pressure and agreed to accept them.

Money was collected from my health insurance card. Money was collected from my debit card. I was shown the door while clutching another card which said *Don't-come-back-for-three-months*.

I wore the new glasses. The long vision was excellent, but as soon as I got home and sat in front of my computer, I knew for certain that the reading portion of the lenses was wrong. I couldn't bear to look at the screen for even a short time.

And so, here we were. They had taken a handsome sum of money from me and left me with glasses that I could not use. I sent their head office an email describing the problem and requesting advice on how best to resolve the situation without recourse to government agencies or lawyers.

This had the desired effect: I received a contrite phone call, an offer of my money back or another assessment, which led to a visit with a fresh young optometrist and, eventually, new glasses. I'm still not sure how I feel about it all, but at least I can read the computer now.

Chapter Twelve

The next step on my Leukaemia journey was a follow-up bone marrow biopsy. The procedure went well, from my point of view; which is to say I don't remember much about it. The same team as last time did the business and they were excellent.

I went to see Dr. Tease about the results. He gave me a short lecture on "cellularity," which is defined as "the degree, quality, or condition of a tissue, as regards the number of its constituent cells that are present."

"As regards the number of its constituent cells that are present" is the clue. Some of the tissue — in this case my bone marrow — wasn't all present. The ragged band on parade were less than a full platoon. The package was a little on the light side and no butcher's thumb would be balancing the scales. There would be no cry of "correct weight" here, nor would there be a steward's enquiry.

Bone marrow normally accounts for 30-70% of total bone structure. I had a mere 10%, which explains my tendency to fall down. I didn't have enough red blood cells escaping the starter's gate and launching themselves into the Punters' Handicap to sustain a full-blooded charge at life.

It took me a long time to absorb the news and pick through the ramifications. One sleepless night several weeks later, the penny dropped. My body was no longer self-regenerating. Without regular blood transfusions, I was a dead man. With regular blood transfusions, I was a dead man, walking.

It was not a cheerful thought at two in the morning. The realisation that I would have to surrender my ambition to scale the Matterhorn was especially galling.

The next time I saw Dr. Tease, I had just the one question.

Will my bone marrow recover and, if so, how quickly will that happen?

His body language said that he suspected the worst, but was taking the line that he had no idea. His facial expressions — a rapid progression through twitch, grimace, and forced smile — agreed, though, to his credit, he maintained excellent eye contact throughout.

It must be tough for a mechanic to have to tell people that, although you worked hard on their car, it was now only fit to be towed to the dump. Same with people, I guess.

Eventually he found the right words. "Time will tell. We hope for the best."

Great!

That meant I was still a chance.

The key indicator, short of yet another bone marrow biopsy, would be the haemoglobin readings gained from occasional blood tests. If the readings fall at a slower rate than previously, my prognosis will be in the positive zone.

It was early days, but the signs had been good. And though I knew my way around now, I was hoping I'd never be admitted to hospital again.

Yeah, right...

Chapter Thirteen

Ahead of my next meeting with Dr. Tease, I had a blood test. My haemoglobin was 84. The Blood Book set up an appointment for me to receive two units of blood on the following Saturday morning at the Oncology Day Centre.

By the time of my meeting with Dr. Tease, I felt like crap. I was weak as tissue paper and coughing relentlessly. Another blood test, a Group & Match[17] needed ahead of Saturday's transfusion, returned a haemoglobin reading of 70.

We met. He did the stethoscope thing, back and front, and decided that I had pneumonia. So he organised for me to be taken to the Emergency Department for the immediate provision of one unit of red blood cells and intravenous antibiotics.

I had a chest x-ray, then was transferred to Ward S5, with a promise that the two units of blood planned for the Oncology Day

---

[17] **Group & Match**: We don't all have the same type of blood. Being given the wrong blood type can result in illness or death, so a lot of work goes into matching your potential transfusion to you. The process of deciding if the donor's blood is compatible with yours is called 'cross-matching.'

I heard the phrases 'Group & Hold' and 'Group & Match' thrown around so much I thought they meant the same thing. A *Group & Hold* is ordered when a patient might, but probably won't, need the blood, as in some surgery. A *Group & Match* is done when blood is more than likely going to be needed, such as in a scheduled transfusion. The difference lies in how much work is done to protect the potential recipient.

Sometimes antibodies to foreign red cell antigens form in a patient's body in response to transfusion. The internationally accepted safeguard used to prevent a transfusion reaction in patients previously transfused within the last three months is that a Group & Match screen expires 72 hours after collection. That rule can be a hassle, but it's designed to save your life, so shut up and be grateful.

Centre on Saturday would be fast-tracked to me in the ward the next day. In my mind, these two units took on a life-and-death status.

Then we learned that the two units of blood I was expecting to receive this day had been cancelled. I don't know for sure who did that or why, nor do I recall anyone ever accepting responsibility for the action.

It was about here that I began to see two things: the first being that the Haematology and Oncology Units in this hospital — while having areas of theoretical overlap — were wildly different in character.

The Oncology Day Centre was calm, efficient, and caring. There were many times over the next week or so when I wished I was in their hands. But I wasn't. Most of the time I was in the hands of people from Haematology, and they made it clear that their level of concern for me was just below their personal interest in recycling fish heads.

The second thing I finally understood was that I would be treated better, much better, as an outpatient of the Oncology Unit than I would as a slab-of-meat inpatient of the Haematology Unit.

I announced that I was leaving: if there was to be no blood transfusion, there was no point in being here.

That triggered the usual storm, with people attempting to browbeat me, or advancing facile arguments in the hope of tricking me into staying.

I had one issue: Where's my blood transfusion?

No answer.

My wife rang the Oncology Day Centre and was able to rescue my programmed transfusion for the next morning. A lone, seventy-one-year-old retiree, with no links to the hospital, managed to do something that a horde of Haematology Registrars and Interns, with all their clout and inside running, had been unable to do.

Or maybe they never wanted to.

The next day, I was given the two units of blood I needed in the Oncology Day Centre by lovely gentle staff. Ahh! The joy of encountering people who care in a large modern hospital.

Chapter Fourteen

About 1:00am a few mornings later, I woke with a heavy, uncontrolled nose bleed. That is to say, blood was gushing from my nose, splashing about my person, and refusing to stop. A box of tissues, applied in clumps in the standard nostril grip for half an hour, was insufficient to impede the flow.

We rang for an ambulance and were assisted by two lovely young men, who took us to the Emergency Department, where a gang of incompetents took turns at shoving needles into my arms.

Sorry to be blunt. I was in a teaching hospital. Most of the staff were young and inexperienced. They had to learn how to get a needle into a vein somewhere. Just not on me. I've been through two full courses of chemotherapy and my veins are mostly AWOL. Even among experienced staff, I'm considered "difficult" and the wiser of those pass me on to the Ninja-grade needle jockeys during the setup for a transfusion.

The key to guiding a length of sharpened steel into a vein is patience and sensitivity. Some people have the fine touch necessary to locate and identify a good vein and some people do not. Practice-makes-perfect can apply, but it remains the case that those with less sensitive fingertips or little patience never really make the grade.

As Clint Eastwood once said[18], "A man's got to know his limitations." Mind you, he went on to say, "Nothing wrong with shooting as long as the right people get shot," which isn't a common view among hospital staff, as they're the ones who'll have to patch up the damage.

---

[18] *Magnum Force* (1973).

Emergency Departments can be places of controlled chaos, with blood and vomit and screaming, or they can be places of calm, even boredom, especially in the wee hours. These quieter times offer an opportunity for practicing the skills of the trade on convenient patients. That approach sometimes reflects the slab-of-meat view of hospital care, in appearance, if not intention.

So here I was, on a boring early morning, requiring needle access for a transfusion, and a crowd had gathered. There were people with ultrasound machines searching for veins, there were people with divining rods, there were people who conducted small animal sacrifices to various gods before leaping into action. A week later, I still had extensive bruising on both arms.

The pinnacle came when the Arrogant Shift Coordinator arrived, announced himself as the World's Greatest needle jockey, and slammed a needle into the inside of my forearm. The pain was unbelievable. I wept uncontrollably for a long time. Eventually even the Arrogant Shift Coordinator started to realise there was a problem. He offered me "pain relief," then slunk away, never to be seen again.

It was four hours before I understood what had happened: the cannula was inserted inside tissue, not a vein. When someone attempted to feed an intravenous antibiotic through it, my wrist expanded like a balloon. Some of the nursing staff grasped what was happening — not many of them, mind — but enough to get it withdrawn.

The real damage was felt by my wife, who was forced to sit and watch me: agony written over my face, weeping silently. She still talks about the experience.

After that, someone competent found a vein and I was given one unit of platelets, one litre of potassium, and a dose of IV antibiotics.

Over a three week period, I had two trips to hospital by ambulance with epistaxis — uncontrolled bleeding from the nose. I was under strict instructions to ring for an ambulance if the bleeding ever lasted more than twenty minutes. I felt like a wuss, but orders is orders.

All the ambos I met were brilliant. Far, far better than most of the Registrars and Interns who followed them.

The worst thing was the bleeding from the eyes, a new experience for me. We were bouncing around in the back of an ambulance on my second trip to hospital. I was looking out the back window at a car that was tailgating us, and thinking, *How stupid do you have to be to tailgate an ambulance* ?

I was clutching my nose with a bunch of tissues in one hand, trying to staunch the flow, when I realised I could no longer see, so I dabbed at my eyes with a tissue in the other hand, and it came away bloody.

I made a joke about it not coming out of my ears yet. It was a surprise to discover that even a weak chuckle from an ambulance officer contains a measure of reassurance.

And I needed a bit of reassurance about then.

It was early Sunday morning and the Emergency Department was full of eager young types. I was covered in blood and therefore looked like an interesting case to discuss with colleagues over breakfast.

They clustered about, all wanting to be a part of things. Made me think of the hospital scene in *Get Shorty* (1995), where the Emergency Department surgeon asks his eager team, "*Okay, who wants to take a crack at wiring Mr. Zimm's jaw?*" Harry Zimm's toes curled; it was not a moment of high confidence for him.

One of the more eager wannabes jumped into fitting a needle in a vein. I quickly figured out that he was faking his way, much like he did — I'm guessing — through Med School.

I could tell instantly that he didn't know what he was doing. There's a certain pain when they do it right and there's a far worse pain when they do it wrong. And this one was wrong.

I endured the pain for a while, wanting for him to succeed and not wanting to be an asshole too quickly, but eventually I had to tell him to get the needle out because that was extremely painful and he obviously had no clue about what he was trying to do.

This dented my popularity with the crowd. The possibility of receiving a public rebuke from a blood-soaked patient threatened the frail masculinity of most of them. They slunk away, feigning a sudden interest in other cases, leaving more air for me to breathe in the little cubicle.

No one volunteered to take another shot at the needle. One woman remained, a nurse called Karen, a gentle, caring soul who — at that moment — was caring for the poor dears who couldn't take honest feedback. Later on, she'd work overtime caring for me.

There were a couple of guys left. They had a chance to do some good and they were ready to try anything. One of them kept making phone calls to an E.N.T. person who did Sunday duty covering all the major hospitals in Adelaide. I was the highest profile E.N.T. drama around, so he was in transit to my hospital.

Meanwhile he was providing advice over the phone. The thing to do here was to get a Rapid Rhino[19] up my nose. And, no, that had nothing to do with African wildlife. It's like a solid foam condom with a pump attached. Once inserted, it is inflated inside the troublesome nostril, building pressure and, hopefully, cutting off

---

[19] **Rhino**: word-forming element meaning "nose, of the nose," from the Greek.

the bleeding. The boys gave that a shot, but I still had blood pouring out my nose, mouth and eyes.

Another phone call. Conclusion? The Rapid Rhino wasn't in far enough. Deflate. Remove. Reinsert much, much, much further inside the nostril.

These guys knew this was going to hurt. They were nice about it, but it was all for my good. I called for a brief Time Out so I could clarify one point.

"Yes?"

"Is swearing allowed?"

There was a brief consultation. Judge's ruling? Yes, swearing was allowed. And we were back to the game.

I was reclining on a cracked, vinyl covered, dentist's chair, with a heap of blood-soaked towels and tissues piled high on my belly. Half my attention was directed toward preventing the tissue box from sliding off the pile, the other half was keeping watch over the boys' latest move.

The junior member kept asking, "Aren't we supposed to wet it first?"

I was thinking, What? The litre of blood flowing past won't moisten it enough for you? Later on, I checked the company video on YouTube[20] and Junior was right. You're supposed to soak it in water for "a full thirty seconds", in order to activate the chemicals in the coating. But in this Emergency Department we didn't have time for reading instructions or soaking stuff or listening to our junior partner.

---

[20] https://www.youtube.com/watch?v=Gn7DX7Bqbtl

Then Jay turned up. He was the travelling Ear, Nose &Throat guy, a young man with movie-star good looks and heaps of confidence. We clashed immediately when he told me to look "up". I eventually determined that what he meant by "up" was "back". Like most doctors, he hated to be corrected over anything and decided that I was "in a bad mood" and had "an attitude problem." Not the start I wanted.

This led into the standard doctor speech about how he's here to help me and how I need to cooperate.

I explained: "If I don't understand what you're saying, I can't cooperate. And I *will* ask questions. The trick with me is to take an extra couple of seconds and explain, *in advance*, what it is you're about to do."

Yes, yes, yes; of course he would explain in advance; but, like many doctors, he had so much stuff going through his head that he had trouble separating things-he-meant-to-say from things-he-actually-said.

Without warning, he jumped into shoving the now-deflated Rapid Rhino as close to my brain as he could get it. The pain was horrible. I applied the licence granted me to swear, and gave voice to my full range of Anglo-Saxon expletives.

You don't know just how far back some of these cavities extend until someone fills one with a half-metre long condom. The pushing stopped. The pain eased. A moment of calm followed.

I mopped the blood from my eyes and opened them. Every spare person in Emergency had congregated at the entrance to my booth to observe the reason for all the swearing. The faces wore sympathetic expressions. I realised that this was due to the enormous amount of blood splashed down my front and resolved to maintain my current appearance for as long as possible.

The calm quickly turned to boredom and the crowd departed.

Jay pulled on a new pair of blue gloves, snapped them at the wrist in an authoritative manner, and advanced on the Rapid Rhino.

The next step was to inflate the thing. He warned me that the increased pressure might hurt and started talking about "pain relief". I would hear *Do-you-want-some-pain-relief* from every person who spoke to me in an official capacity from here on out.

A few quick pumps and we were at four. *Four what*? you ask. No idea, but the numbers went up to ten. That's it; no more than ten. The weigh station of four didn't last long and we were quickly at ten. The increased pressure brought increased pain, but the bleeding dropped to a slow ooze.

Jay went for a walk, taking my file with him. I assume he had updated all the notes by the time he returned. He checked my proboscis. Still no bleeding, other than a slow ooze.

Jay was euphoric. Probably had a long night and was a bit over-tired, but he was thrilled. He was the guy who stopped the bleeding when no one else could. He was the man! His street cred was going to be solid around here for some time to come.

He high-fived me and told me what a good bloke I was. We agreed that things didn't start well. We tussled, I said, but you won on points. He was pleased/embarrassed, and brushed my suggestion aside.

We discussed my pain level. I told him I was grateful this wasn't *Spinal Tap*[21] with Nigel Tufnel's amplifier going all the way to eleven. Ten was painful enough.

Then I twigged. This wasn't *Spinal Tap*, this was *Men in Black* (1997). We had Jay, the main character; we had Karen, that's Kay;

---

[21] The 1984 mockumentary *This Is Spinal Tap*. One of the best-known scenes from the film involves the band member Nigel Tufnel explaining how their amplifiers go all the way up to eleven, not just ten, like for most other bands.

and Jay had the little light-thingy. He was saying to me, "Look at the light," as he approached my other nostril.

I told him I knew we were in *Men in Black* and now he was going to flash me with the light-thingy and erase my memory. But Jay said, No. He wanted me to remember, so I could tell the E.N.T. Registrar tomorrow how he tussled with me, *mano e mano*, and won on points.

Sometimes these things are important to young men. Me, I kept looking about for the little talking dog, but I never saw him.

By now, I was busting for a leak. I got up to go to the toilet.

"Turn right, across the open space to that corridor, then along the corridor to the second door on your left."

Okay.

I broke into a slow-motion shuffle and was making good time, part of the way to the open space, when one of the Emergency Department nurses stopped me and asked, "Do you normally walk with a stick?"

This was unexpected. I considered things a moment, then leaned toward him, patted myself on the left shoulder and said, "I normally have a parrot[22] on this shoulder." The guy was coming to the end of a night shift and had reached the *Everything-Is-Funny* stage. He began to giggle and couldn't stop.

---

[22] For a while after I collapsed in the street and was stitched up in the Emergency Department, I sported an impressive looking scar above my left eye, with large black stitches on prominent display. As this attracted attention wherever I went, I developed a patter about obtaining a **parrot** to sit on my shoulder and said that, maybe, I could go into a new line of business. Instead I found that government regulations restricted ownership of Australian wildlife to people of good character, so my putative new career never really blossomed. I must have had the possibility still in view at this time.

I resumed my shuffle.

An older guy, a hillbilly type, tall and thin, got up from a chair in the waiting area and shaped up like one of those Boxing Tent blokes who used to travel around the various country Fairs, making money from beating up drunks.

I'd never seen him before. I guess that the blood sprayed over me from nostrils to knees reminded him of the Good Old Days.

I adopted a similar stance to his. He was grinning at maximum grin. I jiggled closer, paused, and said, "Ya shoulda seen the other guy."

This had him laughing so hard he had to rest amidst his family entourage, the youngest of whom was sitting, cross-legged, down the end, playing the fiddle. The tune sounded familiar, but I couldn't place it.

Chapter Fifteen

After that I was moved to Ward Q5. This was a Crimean War-style place, with lots of blokes crammed in together, with curtains around them. How many, I couldn't say, but I was in bed 17. We were crammed so close together that I might as well have been in the same bed as the guy on the left. As it was, he spent half the night holding my hand and muttering something about still respecting me in the morning.

I didn't sleep a wink.

Next morning, I had that wide-awake-but-exhausted feeling. I was also constipated. This eventually lead to a moment of pure transcendence, as the main bolus moved slowly past the point-of-no-return, leaving me with a sense of relief such as money cannot buy.

Following that first trip to the local convenience, I had a feeling of internal collapse, one coinciding with my suddenly vacant gut. At least, it felt 'suddenly vacant.' That's misleading, of course. Much remained, but it was soft and pliable and currently considering a career in public life.

I'm talking about something fertile, something with a mind of its own. You may countermand, over-rule, invalidate, even retract any base gut decision, but once that decision has led to the missile being moved into the firing chamber, it's time to be somewhere else. In my case, that would be: (a) out of bed, (b) disconnected from an infusion line, and (c) hotfooting it to the nearest toilet.

It was not as simple as it sounds.

I was already butt-clenching in fear as I blocked the flow of the drip and disconnected the line. Then I was away in my patented *Old-Man-Slow-Shuffle*, praying grimly as I went, that the destination would be vacant and, well, *clean* would be nice.

I never attempted the Ewan McGregor prayer[23] for *"a massive pristine convenience, brilliant gold taps, virginal white marble, a seat carved from ebony, a cistern full of Chanel No. 5, and a flunky handing me pieces of raw silk toilet roll."* No, no, no. On the inside I was screaming, "Please, God, get me to the dunny[24] on time."

The second last corner, that's where I came undone. My quick release of the clench in order to gain a better grip, that was a mistake.

I felt the slip. I felt the splat, as my new Jocks took a full load for the team. I felt the overwhelming sense of shame, just as I burst into a huge, square room with a small throne in the far corner, rolled up my combination of back and front gowns, eased down an amazingly heavy pair of Jocks and sat. There followed an explosion which sprayed the bowl. It shook the building, or... okay, it just shook me.

I was able to separate myself from the bulging Jocks without doing any further damage to anything. Them, they had to go, and go they did, into a convenient trash receptacle. That left me bare-assed, shaken, and experiencing a series of gut explosions which added layers to the rich tapestry building in the bowl.

All in all, another small incident never reported to management.

---

[23] From *Trainspotting* (1996). Renton is cleaning up his drug habit. Long-term heroin use leads to constipation; withdrawal can result in the body reversing the process, sometimes in dramatic fashion.
[24] Australian slang, meaning 'a toilet.' The word comes from the Scots' *dunnekin* meaning an 'earth closet, (outside) privy' — from *dung* + *ken* 'house'. Originally referred to outside facilities, but now extends to any toilet.

Once I was fully relieved, re-gowned and returned to my curtained bed, the Ear Nose & Throat (E.N.T.) registrar arrived, with entourage.

I have always found those moments disconcerting, when I am ripped from private reverie into full arena entertainment by the abrupt wrenching of a curtain.

The realisation that I was under scrutiny by a small horde of white-coated people, most of whom were clutching clipboards and displaying fixed smiles, triggered a sense of vague schoolboy guilt: I was sure I must have been doing something wrong, but couldn't quite remember what it was.

One of the Fixed Smiles made a short announcement, invoking the name, rank and serial number of the more important crowd members, but as I had trouble locating which Fixed Smile it was doing the speaking, I missed out on the details.

It seemed rude to demand that they do it again — preferably with the speaker waving a white handkerchief, or at least clutching a Talking Pillow[25] — merely to assist my comprehension.

I had first encountered this E.N.T. registrar a few days earlier, while in a different bed in a different ward, and she had given me loads of friendly, helpful, caring advice. Now, in what passed for light-hearted badinage, mostly for the benefit of her admiring hangers-on, she admonished me for failing to take that advice, epistaxis being a major element on her no-no list; but had I been listening…?

We eased past the compulsory Humour-in-hospital section and got to the point. The Rapid Rhino had to come out. This wasn't a task she would bother herself with, but she had a young intern

---

[25] **Talking Pillow:** One technique for regulating a group discussion: the person holding the designated item (pillow) is the only one allowed to speak.

with her who needed practice at the subtle art of ripping something out of a patient's head.

The rest of the circus moved on.

The intern remained. She was a gangly, eager-to-please young woman, for whom nothing was too much trouble.

I was sitting in a chair next to the bed at the time. Most of my hospital admissions have been to chairless locations, ones which left me with only the side of a traditional iron hospital bed, with girders attached for bed-tilting purposes. These required me to sit with my legs draped over an iron bar and my feet dangling high above the floor. That's perfectly comfortable for the first ten seconds or so, then the various iron bars started to cut into my legs, first numbing, then gouging them.

My major recent advance in hospital survival skills was to learn to ask for a chair at the moment of admission, a technique which has been rewarded every time.

Gangly Intern approached the Rapid Rhino. This required her to flex, bend, then double over, before she could reach down to the target. Her back creaked; a joint made a popping sound; the manoeuvre reminded me of a cherry-picker suffering hydraulic failure and experiencing a powerless fade to ground level.

I suggested that I could relocate to make this easier, but she was a saint. Nothing was too much trouble, she was here to help.

The Rapid Rhino had, over the last twenty-four hours — under pressure from being pumped up to ten — adhered to the nasal lining. A quick wrench should be enough to remove an entire layer of flesh and start the epistaxis problem all over again.

I still had my neighbour's promise to respect me in the morning rolling around in my head. The thought of another day in bed 17 promised more excitement than I could bear.

I called for a halt to proceedings and clambered back onto the bed, moving the Rapid Rhino a metre closer to the eyeline of Gangly Intern. She straightened up. Her back joint made another popping sound.

This new arrangement seemed to agree with her, for she conjured a special looking case from the floor and laid it on the bed. It opened to reveal a machine with a long fibre-optic cable attached, such as would have been acceptable in any modern day, hi-tech, heist movie.

The business end of the cable was introduced briefly into my empty nostril for, I assume, testing purposes. A full set of green lights there led to a forced probe past the now deflated Rapid Rhino in the other nostril. This brought back memories of Jay, the Emergency Department team, and swearing.

The probe didn't last long, but it gave full value as a tunnelling device. The fibre-optic cable was replaced by a thin tube attached to a plastic bottle, which released a liquid solvent into the tunnel. A quick squirt, then all was withdrawn so we could await the outcome.

Gangly Intern disappeared into the bowels of the hospital. I half-lay, propped up in the bed, and waited. A couple of hours drifted by, as I listened from behind my security curtain to the sounds of an overcrowded ward shrugging off excess patients and gearing up for new arrivals.

I was beginning to worry, when the curtain burst open.

Gangly Intern had returned, equipped with a bag of plumber's tools. She selected a small pair of pliers and went to work with those on the Rapid Rhino.

A gentle twist, a tug, and a great length of blood-stained cloth unrolled from my nose, a bit like Krusty the Clown extracting an endless string of coloured flags from his mouth.

There was a shared moment as we, together, braced for a spray of blood, but all was still.

Wow, the sense of relief! Gangly Intern seemed more pleased than myself. She stood awhile, admiring her success, then brought out her fibre-optic trick pack for a rerun at close quarter internal examination. I thought this probably unnecessary, but I was grateful for Gangly's gentle work and let her have her way.

"There's still a large clot in there," she announced.

"Oh?"

Gangly produced a two-pronged length of stainless steel from her bag of plumber's tools. This she introduced into my nostril, thrusting and nipping at an unseen growth. In advance after advance, she failed to obtain the hold she wanted, so she repositioned her light source and her lengthy grippers and tried again. And again. It was like a lion-tamer, armed with chair and whip, keeping a growling young lion at bay.

The combination of duelling hardware and pressured tissue triggered a sense of panic. Something was beginning to move around back there and I pictured a throat *Alien* bursting out of its birth sac.

I growl-waved her off and Gangly withdrew. I gave a gulp, made a snort, unleashed a strangled choking sound, moved into a raucous throat-clearing, gave a frightened squawk, then a huge polyp of dried blood burst from my mouth, landed in a towel I was holding and lay there, looking up at us. It was too big to hold in one hand.

I expected Gangly Intern to round off the moment by thrusting a stake through its heart, but instead she stood there, smiling softly, admiring our collective work.

Just one more satisfying day at the office.

Chapter Sixteen

She was typical: twenty-four, short, slim, pretty, smug, and absolutely confident in her God-given powers as a nurse. She asked me the classic hospital question:

"Do you have any pain?"

The question was asked in a gentle, caring manner, itself proof positive that I had arrived in the Land of Happiness and Health.

Do you have any pain?

I suppose that, back when I was twenty-four, if I'd had any pain, the area would have been highlighted by a throbbing red light. Now that I'm sixty-three, and blessed with varying levels of asthma, arthritis, diabetes, sinusitis, low haemoglobin, high cholesterol, sore throat, gravitational eczema, myelodysplastic syndrome, Charcot foot, back pain, nose bleeds, autonomic neuropathy, nausea, heartburn, constipation, grumbling appendix, bladder problems, difficulty with swallowing, difficulty with blood pressure control, and an irregular heart beat, a single throbbing red light for every point of discomfort would turn me into a glowing Kreemorian Fangor Beast[26], scarier than what any Smug Nurse could deal with.

Do you have any pain?

The truth is, most of us old people don't talk about it. We don't think about it. We operate under the unwritten provisions of *Old-Person-Getting-Through-The-Day* etiquette.

---

[26] **Kreemorian Fangor Beast**: From *Galaxy Quest* (1999). Tim Allen: "You know, guys, I had a late night with a Kreemorian Fangor Beast, so I'm gonna just shut my eyes for a little bit. Go on, I'm listening to everything you say."

This might be the last day for one of us, so the other party doesn't want to waste your last minutes by banging on with endless, unimportant trivia, as that would seem rude. To have to get up and say at the funeral: "I wasted this poor beggar's last day by listing my ailments in lexicographical order for about two hours. He seemed interested at first, then his pallor changed, he gagged a couple of times, and fell to the floor. The ambulance guys said there was nothing they could do."

Do you have any pain?

This is the moment when my head sags into my hands, a short script of possible responses flashes before my eyes. I conduct a brief struggle for self-control and a measure of social acceptance.

"Yes, we have no bananas."

No, that's not it.

"Nah, no pain."

A bald-faced lie, my favourite kind.

"Waddaya think, ya dopey woman? I hurt all over."

Possibly not polite enough.

"Yeah, no, some."

I plump for the vague option, in the hope Smug Nurse will be happy to fill in whatever details are currently most socially-acceptable.

"Would you like some pain relief?"

I started to think about the subject of pain and pain relief while awaiting discharge from the hospital. There was another guy ahead of me in the queue, a man in his thirties, from the bush[27], who had been in the ward for a few weeks. I was unable to avoid hearing his anxious questions about obtaining the same quantities of oxycodone[28] he had become accustomed to receive in hospital.

"Oh, we can't let you have that much. It's legal while you're in hospital, but illegal outside. We'll give you a prescription for the legal dose when you go home."

Wow. This poor man had been set up by the hospital for a bout of opiate withdrawal just as he had to adjust to the reality of being back in the bush, at a distance from any medical support. I don't know what he went through or how things worked out for him, but I know I never wanted to be in his position.

Would you like some pain relief?

No, thanks, I'll be fine.

---

[27] **The bush**: An all-encompassing term for the Australian countryside. From the earliest days of European settlement, it's been a question of "the city or the bush," with the city winning out by a wide margin. I've met a few Poms who pointed out that most Australians live less than one hundred miles from the sea, as if this were a national character flaw. I tell them that no Brit lives more than eighty miles from the sea, and that the whacking great desert at the centre of the wide, brown land has something to do with our choices.

[28] **Oxycodone hydrochloride** is an opioid analgesic. It is a depressant drug, in the same class as alcohol, cannabis and heroin. I knew it as *hillbilly heroin*, a name not recognised by the nurses who tried to administer it to me during my last hospital admission. The media in Australia have recently discovered its role as a gateway drug to many other addictions and abuses.

Chapter Seventeen

Prior to my second bout of chemotherapy, a small lump had appeared on the side of my nose. During the chemo, it shrank down to almost nothing, and I dismissed it. A year later, it suddenly reappeared and grew at an alarming rate.

This led to a visit to a plastic surgeon and another bout of Day Surgery. I wasn't at my prettiest when I left.

The surgery required a graft, which was held in place by twenty-six stitches. The graft came from the side of my neck, a long gash which required another sixteen stitches, which left me looking as though I'd done poorly in a fencing bout, perhaps as the hapless victim of a swashbuckling Douglas Fairbanks, or Errol Flynn, or maybe Mandy Patinkin.

The biopsy taken at the time came back with the bad news that we were dealing with a squamous cell carcinoma, the more aggressive form of skin cancer. They had failed to get all of it and I was now required to undergo thirty days of radiotherapy in the hope of clearing things up.

The radiotherapy was not a lengthy process, with most of my time each day being chewed up in the waiting room.

Once my turn was announced, I was herded into a small room with a large machine and a narrow bed on a railway track. This was not a place for a quick bit of rumpy-pumpy after hours. I always felt I was balancing on a thick knife edge, high above the stage, with the circus-master extolling my courage to the audience, while emphasizing the dangers inherent in performing this trick.

The two people present — radiation commandos, both trained to deal forcibly with skittish patients — were also programmed to be hyper-encouraging. While I reclined, searched for non-existent finger grips on the side of the knife and hung on, they waited for my belly to stop jiggling.

During this stage, they ran through every encouraging thought they could muster: How well I was doing, how well I was looking, how far I'd come (*Only twenty-two more visits to go, whoo-hoo!*), or how close to the weekend we were — time off from this routine being as welcome to them as it was to me.

They tried to distract me with questions about what I did last night, what I plan for this afternoon or evening or weekend. I found the process bordering on the patronising and responded by complaining about my radiation disappointment.

Everyone knows from the movies that when a bloke is exposed to this much radiation, he develops super-powers and has to go out and buy a costume and a cape. I've always fancied the cape, if not the public display of brightly-coloured underwear, so I was disappointed to be getting nothing: not the speeding bullet, not the locomotive, not the tall buildings, nothing.

On one occasion, a nurse who previously worked in the Radiotherapy unit of a large research hospital told me how they used to give leukaemia to mice, then expose each one to a different level of radiation, just to see what would happen. One day, a lab assistant carrying a tray of these radioactive mice managed to drop it. The mice scattered and were never recovered.

It's the stuff of legend that cleaners have reported seeing, late at night, glowing mice, scurrying away into the distance. The story was intended to cheer me up, but I kept thinking that at least the mice got to glow in the dark; you just know they'd be popular at mouse parties. Me, I got nothing.

So, we ran out of anecdotes, the jiggling midriff subsided; it was time to get started. A sheet of Heat Shrink plastic was spread across my head. This had already been treated to conform to the shape of my face. It did an excellent job of covering my nose and mouth: I was unable to breathe and began to asphyxiate.

The only thing that kept me from breaking out in panic-stricken flailing, with a burst of the invective popular among goat-herders in the old country, was the knowledge that I had close to two minutes before I passed out. *Stuff I learned in Boy Scouts.*

While I was counting down the first minute, and pondering the super-powers I would now never know, someone went to work with a sharp Texta pen, marking dots on and around my nose. These provided a grid, visible on camera to the machine operator, who would be huddled in safety behind five tonnes of lead at the time of launching my next not-quite-lethal dose of radiation.

The human face is not an easy place to do graffiti. Most operators established a stable position by resting their hand, first on one eyeball, then on the other. I found this painful, but my moaning and quiet sobbing brought no relief. Once the dots were in place, the plastic was removed and, in a whistling gasp, I resumed my breathing.

The idea behind my treatment was to focus the nuclear rays so that they built a concentration in the cartilage in the middle of my nose, where the cancer had taken hold, and lay waste — in the style of Attila the Hun — anything resembling a squamous cell carcinoma.

One of the peculiarities of radiation is that it likes open space, which meant that, if left vacant, my nostrils would fill with playful nuclear power, which would bound about in a game resembling *Red Rover*, while the internal surfaces were stripped bare of useful skin.

To get around this problem, sharpened bamboo sticks were wrapped in gauze, coated with a thin layer of Vaseline, and thrust into the cavities. I resembled a walrus, especially when I tried to speak.

All nose-breathing ceased. I was reduced to mouth-gasping, a process which dried the tissues and left my mouth like something resembling a clay pan baked in the sun in Death Valley.

I learned to pre-empt this problem by slipping a cough lolly into my mouth before reclining on the knife edge. The mentholated sweet promoted the production of saliva, but created another problem — the fear of accidentally swallowing, or inhaling, the medicinal candy. Fear of choking helped focus the mind and kept me from thinking too much about nose bleeds and the spectre of epistaxis.

The vinyl-covered pillows were adjusted; my head was lifted, tilted and angled. To keep me from moving, I was bound in position with a roll of duct tape. As the first length was stretched against my forehead, the slap of the tape released a wave of cold sweat across my face. This caused me to flinch, which was good, because the next step was the placement of lead pieces on my scrunched-up eyes. These half-kilo weights were another source of pain and left me with flat eyeballs and distorted vision for some time afterwards.

The two radiation commandos murmured numbers to one another, read from a checklist, reviewed the markings and, after a quick confirmation that they had the right victim bound and gagged, they scarpered from the blast zone.

I lay perfectly still and thought of film clips I'd seen of nuclear explosions and the aftermath of Hiroshima and Nagasaki. A light, bright enough to penetrate the lead shields over my eyes, filled the room. I listened for Spielberg's five tones inviting me aboard the mothership or the sound associated with the jump to hyperspace, but all I heard was myself, sobbing softly.

Eventually the light went out. I continued to lie still, awaiting the return of my captors. They were not in a hurry to run into the residual radiation washing about the room, but eventually risked it. I heard the cheery cry of "All done," and wrestled the weights from my eyes.

Some time was expended in unravelling the duct tape, removing the sharpened bamboo from my nostrils, and generally clearing away the evidence of what had just happened to me.

The radiation commandos clustered about me as I tried to sit up. They were solicitous of my well-being and careful to keep me from plunging to the floor. I suspect that such an event would result in radiation leaking from any head wound.

The usual finale to all this was a ceremonial washing to remove the Maori-like face markings prior to my return to the outside world, but they quickly learned that I was eager to escape and they stopped bothering.

I emerged into bright sunshine and walked a dozen blocks to my bus stop. Along the way, I passed a homeless refuge. I could tell it was a homeless refuge because the street was lined with people in various stages of dissolution, who engaged one another in intense discussion, not always of a common subject.

The seat of the closest bus shelter was occupied with two or three people, and fifteen or twenty bottles in plastic bags. I didn't bother with it; I was headed to the next stop.

The first time, as I shuffled up — a fat man in a clean shirt, waddling defencelessly through a sea of people who knew hard times and understood the need for a bit of initiative — I sparked ideas in the crowd. Small light bulbs lit up over their heads: *Here's a soft touch for the price of a cask of wine.* A couple of them seized the moment and advanced on me with a welcoming cry of, "How's it goin', bro'?"

I peered at them from behind my Maori mask, pulled out my deep voice and said, "Nostrovia[29]!" — the Russian equivalent of "Cheers."

I have no idea what this word conveyed to them, but I could see the cogs turning as they wondered: *What did he say? What does that mean? Why did he say that to us?* And so on.

They were still in the questioning stage when I had moved well past them and was gone. Perhaps the Russian mafia has been here before. Who knows. Regardless, after that first time, I had no further trouble with any of the locals.

---

[29] **Nostrovia** is an English mispronunciation of the Russian word *Na Zdorovie*. The word is also used in Poland. I don't know who got to it first. It is commonly believed that *Na Zdorovie* is used as a drinking toast.

Chapter Eighteen

I had a blood test at my G.P.'s offices about 2:00pm on Friday 10 February. At about 4:30pm the same day, I received a phone call from the Blood Book telling me I needed to come in for a transfusion.

I was astonished and said so. That was impossibly quick. The woman at the Blood Book replied that the "stars must have aligned for once."

In the past, I have waited up to 48 hours before receiving pathology results. I hadn't expected to hear before the Monday and started to think someone must have had a supply of pixie dust to make that kind of magic happen.

An appointment was set for me at the Oncology Day Centre (ODC) at 9:00am on the next day. I arrived early, the first of what turned out to be a larger than normal Saturday morning crowd.

During the search for a vein that would accept a cannula, my needle jockey and I engaged in a discussion of the ordinary workings of the Blood Book and the blinding efficiency of the O.D.C. in this particular case.

I was suggesting this was out of the *Twilight Zone*, when someone announced that there was no Group & Match for me.

This provoked some hard thinking and a revisit of the steps that had brought me to this place. The physical Blood Book was located — actually a large red folder. I am normally barred from so much as a glimpse of the sacred text, so I watched proceedings with interest. After a short ceremony involving white robes, incense, and Latin chanting, my page was opened on the altar.

A cold breeze moved through the room. Candles flickered. A distant choir burst into *Exsultate justi*.
> *Laudamus te, laudamus !*
> *Exsultate, justi, in Domino;*
> *Exsultate in Domino.*

The build-up was nerve-wracking, worse than the pre-match jostling at a football match.

And this I learned: every person listed in the Blood Book has their computer record checked twice a day by some Lucky Staff Member (LSM), to see if a blood test has taken place, with an examination of relevant parameters in those cases that do pop up.

Yes, twice a day.

And it came to pass, about 4:00pm on Friday the 10th of February, that our LSM, after a day spent staring at a computer screen in a search for a date starting with a "10," suddenly spotted one. On my record. With a haemoglobin result below the trigger level. Our LSM gave a whoop and a short holler, opened negotiations with a person who would be working on the Saturday, and shoe-horned me onto their roster. Another triumph for diligence; a good day's work all round.

Trouble was, the record in question was from 10 January, not 10 February. Yes, Virginia, there is a weakness in the system; it involves any compound of fatigue and human error. Or, in this case, the miraculous juxtaposition of an unexamined blood test and an old record.

Saturday mornings at the ODC are conducted by a skeleton staff. The skeletons on this day[30] were of that rare, above-the-average, problem-solving class. They went to work on the problem; rang

---

[30] Jenny B and Stacey, no less. Two of the finest ninja-grade needle jockeys I've ever met.

the pathology firm, obtained the relevant numbers from Friday's test, took a blood sample from me, talked to the secret Blood Supply, Wizard Unit — *eye of newt, and toe of frog, wool of bat, and tongue of dog* — and arranged for the sample to be turned into a unit of blood.

And it only took two hours. By 12:30pm, I was being prodded and told to wake up, for lo and behold, I could go home.

It was only one face-saving unit of blood, so I knew I'd be back there sooner than normal. Still, it was an interesting morning.

Chapter Nineteen

I developed a cough. A persistent cough. A different cough to those that had gone before. I thought it related to my asthma. Dr. Tease didn't like it. It had been fifteen months since my last CT scan; now he called for another.

So here I was, back where it all started, sitting in the broom closet with the two doors. The big difference this time was in personnel. An older nurse with a serious No Nonsense manner, and a touch of menace, was in charge.

She was brusque. She was brisk. She was blunt.

"Just lose the shirt, the shoes and the braces, then get up on the table."

I obeyed.

I didn't shout *"Jawohl !"*[31] or click my heels, or salute. I just obeyed. I didn't want to provoke her.

Barefoot, bare chested, and clutching at my sagging trousers, I waddled over to the familiar white donut. The nurse attempted to assist me aboard, making contact with the coldest hands I'd ever encountered.

"Oooh. Cold hands!"

"Cold heart, too."

---

[31] My wife is studying German at the moment; I can't stop her. I hear her lessons in the background and help out by shouting *"Raus! Schnell! Achtung!"* and other movie-German expressions that come to mind as I pass by.

I'd been thinking something along those lines myself, and was about to be cheeky, when I noticed that Cold Heart had disappeared. She was back to passing instructions via the moving-talking machine.

The donut hummed. The tray settled into position. The machine said, "Take a deep breath and hold it."

I was reflecting that I wouldn't be here if I could take a deep breath, when the tray bolted for the finish line. Midway I experienced a muscle spasm in my back and a minor coughing fit in my front.

The resultant contortions meant the take was ruined and we would have to go again.

Back we went. The machine repeated its instructions. The tray gave a shudder and off we went on our short journey. I coughed. My back twinged. And another take was ruined.

This time Cold Heart came into the room to talk me through the situation, as she saw it.

"It's only nine seconds. Just hold your breath for NINE SECONDS. Can you do that?" Her tone of voice added the unspoken addendum: *You blithering idiot* !

I was thinking that maybe we were about to cast our feelings into words, and was toying with "You brazen hussy" — a popular rebuke among the nuns when I was in elementary school — as a possible opening bid, but she didn't say any more.

I was left feeling vulnerable and offered up the plea of disability. "I've got a muscle spasm in my back." I contorted in an effort to demonstrate the truth of my claim.

Cold Heart slapped me. Across my naked shoulder. Hard.

The shock of the moment caused me to freeze. In that state of suspended animation, the scan was completed, contortion- and cough-free.

Cold Heart reappeared. I don't know if it's my silhouette or the fact that so many parts of me jiggle, but I have noticed a pattern of concern among nurses. They worry about my dismount technique.

"How do you normally get off the bed?"

"I put my feet over the edge and pray that the rest of me follows."

I put my feet over the edge. The rest of me followed, like a slinky working its way down stairs. Once the full complement of disks had clicked into place, I braced my shoulders, fixed a manly expression to my face, and waddled back to the broom closet with my head held high.

No one spoke.

The one thing Gene Kelly[32] and I have in common is the motto: "Dignity. Always dignity."

---

[32] One of Gene Kelly's greatest roles was in *Singin' in the Rain* (1952), during which he recounted a largely fictitious version of his life story to a red carpet media interviewer, and three times claimed that his life had been marked by 'Dignity. Always dignity.'

Chapter Twenty

The motto would be tested in the days ahead, as I developed something called "C.C.F." That's Congestive Cardiac Failure[33] to you, or shortness of breath, excessive tiredness and ugly swollen ankles to me.

I have discovered that everybody in medical circles can recognise C.C.F. ankles at a glance. Their reactions range from shock, through horror, to mouth-clutching dismay. If you're the only person in the room who doesn't know what it is they're reacting to, the experience can be disturbing.

I was booked in to see my G.P. for an annual flu shot on the Tuesday after Easter. He took one look at the ugly ankles, refused me a flu shot, and shunted me off to hospital with a note requesting a review of my symptoms.

I spent the rest of the day in the Emergency Department, where the usual routine of small crowds asking questions in relay commenced. I was placed on a nebuliser, had a chest x-ray, an electrocardiogram (E.C.G.) and some blood tests. This filled the hours from 11:00am to 2:00pm. By then I was not only hungry, but in danger of falling into hypoglycaemia.

No food was offered to me. I knew from experience that this Emergency Department wasn't attuned to the food

---

[33] **Congestive cardiac failure**, also called chronic heart failure (CHF), is an ongoing condition in which the heart muscle is weakened and can't pump as well as it normally does. The main pumping chambers of the heart (the ventricles) become larger or thicker, and either can't contract (squeeze) or can't relax as well as they should. This triggers fluid retention, particularly in the lungs, legs and abdomen. The major causes include coronary heart disease, hypertension, cardiomyopathy and other heart diseases.

requirements of diabetic patients, but the building had a Kiosk, run by volunteers, where I could probably score a salad roll. So I bundled up my leather shoulder bag over my scrawny old hospital gown and set sail for Food Heaven, heavy breathing as I went, much like a tramp steamer under a full load.

The sight of a fat diabetic, lumbering noisily in the direction of the food that could hold him back from a coma, was too much for some of the nursing staff. They formed a rugby scrum to block my way and we entered into a fifteen minute confrontation.

The gist of it was that they didn't approve of my attempting to obtain food on my own terms, whereas I didn't approve of being left foodless and helpless, and was determined to eat something that would allow me to see out the day while still conscious.

One of the nurses had a sudden epiphany: she had the gift of being able to locate food. This led to a series of earnest declarations about what could be done on my behalf.

When pushed for details, she thrust her shoulders back, swished her hair, and like an auctioneer greeting an opening bid, announced that she could provide me with a … curried … egg … sandwich.

For the benefit of anyone who did not grow up in Australia in the nineteen-sixties, I need to explain a few things. In those days, kids were given their lunches to take to school with them. The well-heeled might have had a fancy tin box, but most of us carried ours in new-fangled plastic containers. These lay about the classroom for hours before lunch and, in the warmer weather, developed a spectacular adjunct of noxious gas.

Anything involving fish could be unpleasant, but the king of the appetite crushers was the humble curried egg sandwich.

This universal experience gave rise to the standard question asked whenever someone dropped an air biscuit — also known as farting, blowing off, or shooting the shit breeze —*Who opened their lunch box*? The only equivalent, and something that suggests a similar degree of distastefulness, was the Australian classic: *Who cut the dog in half*?

To be offered a curried egg sandwich to eat is, to me, the equivalent of being invited to a Syrian gas party. You might not die, but you'll be wishing you had.

I declined the offer and recommenced my journey. After several rest stops along the way, I made it to the Kiosk. Most of the good stuff had sold out, but I acquired an apple and cinnamon cake which I ate rather quickly.

On my return after 3:00pm that afternoon, I found a curried egg sandwich sitting in the middle of the bed.

Okay. Someone had taken offence and wanted to make a point. I decided to let it go, but started to wonder why I was hanging around with these people.

A junior cardiologist arrived to give me the results of the E.C.G. It seems I had experienced a secret heart attack, which is to say, a heart attack that I didn't notice. Diabetics often don't experience pain when having a heart attack, but the body releases a protein called *troponin*[34] into the blood, a dead giveaway.

There was more they didn't know than what there was they did know. They needed an echocardiogram and an angiogram. Apparently the first could happen that afternoon, while the second needed me to fast from midnight of whatever day it was going to take place. Angiograms were in high demand and I might have to wait.

---

[34] **Troponins** are a family of proteins found in skeletal and heart muscle fibres that produce muscular contraction. Troponin tests measure the level of cardiac-specific troponin in the blood to help detect heart injury.

His duty done, the young man now departed. I remained and, with my legs jiggling over the side of the bed, ticked off another four hours. In that time, nothing happened. No tests. No echocardiogram. No friendly visits. No results. No prognosis. No invitations to arm-wrestling, wallaby-racing or wombat-fighting. No food. No nothing.

It was a bleak time. I had started the day expecting a flu shot and, having failed to acquire that, had managed to join the ranks of the unwelcome. There was only one option left: I had to go home. I got dressed, signed the paperwork and headed for the door.

As usual, any suggestion of a patient wanting to leave was greeted with outrage. After hours of silence, I was now the recipient of shouted expressions of concern. It seems that, if I wasn't careful, I could die of a heart attack on the bus!

I continued walking, head held high.

Dignity. Always dignity.

Chapter Twenty-One

That night I ate crisp chicken and vegetable spring rolls, ones I had made myself and stored in the freezer. They were nutritious, delicious, crunchy: nothing like hospital food.

I slept the sleep of the just. Next morning, refreshed and eager, I was working on my computer when the phone rang. It was the Blood Book. They had results from one of yesterday's tests; my haemoglobin was down to 90. I was due for a transfusion, but they were overloaded.

What to do?

Here was I, a recent inpatient, with an unresolved medical condition. Maybe I could go back to the Emergency Department, have a Group & Match test and receive my transfusion there?

There was some back-and-forthing, with Dr. Tease playing a role in the background. The upshot of it all was that I would return to the Emergency Department, where I would be handled by the crack 'B' Team, instead of yesterday's lumbering 'A' division.

The 'B' Team were young, fast, efficient, noisy and obviously thrilled to be doing this job. They were also slightly on edge in anticipation of the arrival of a helicopter carrying victims of a major road crash out in the bush. They had my notes from the previous day, so it was all straightforward.

A cannula, a blood sample, an injection of diuretic, then it was off to the holding bay with me, while they waited for a bed to be freed up.

Eventually I was shifted to Bed 11 in ward 6A. This was in a corner, with a curtain drawn around it; a cramped small space. I was chained to an E.C.G. machine on one side and to an oxygen supply on the other. Three tiny steps in one direction, and another three back the other way, were my limit. I felt like a dog that has been restrained for everyone's protection.

When I arrived, the ward was empty. Over the next twenty-four hours it filled up, mostly with farmers. The thing these people have in common — apart from heart attacks and the ownership of large tracts of the wide, brown land — is a fondness for turning their TV up so loud you can hear it in North Korea. I think it's their way of keeping the sheep in the back paddock company.

Last year I encountered a Korean nurse, Kwang, in this ward. He was wonderful. If we were picking sides for the International Nursing Uphill Slalom and Etiquette competition, he'd be the first person I voted for. He was kind, he was gentle, the guy knew his *kimchi*. He was also competitive. We got onto the subject of food and I told him of my worst ever food experience.

We were at a wedding in Malaysia — one of those endless-number-of-courses Chinese banquets — when the waiters brought around white plates. In the middle of the white plate was a tiny baby octopus, all pink and shiny. There was no sauce. There was no lettuce or other greens. There was only baby octopus.

Shiny. Pink.

I looked at Baby a long time. I thought many things, but was unable to bring myself to thrust my fork into his pink and shiny body.

(Yes, I had a fork. We had asked the waiter to take the two pieces of wood away and hide them, so no one noticed that the ignorant *gweilo*[35] were handicapped in the Comparative Cultures Eating Stakes.)

---

[35] **Gweilo**: A common Cantonese slang term for Westerners.

Eventually a waiter came and, on a nod from me, took Baby away, still shiny and whole.

As I finished the story, Kwang nodded wisely. Then he told us that in Korea, baby octopus were served on special occasions. The difference being that Korean baby octopus were still alive. The trick to eating them safely was to take them into your mouth and instantly bite the head from the body. If you delayed, the octopus would make itself at home and lock down your lips, tongue and the wobbly bit above your throat, using the suckers on various arms, and slowly kill you.

I still don't know if Kwang was winding me up, but I have lost plenty of sleep since to fanciful reimaginings of the baby-octopus-in-the-mouth scenarios.

Back in heart attack country, amidst the roaring television sets, I started to catch up on daytime TV, with shows like *The Bald and the Pretty*, *The Long and the Resting*, and *I'm A Clot Get Me Out of Here* blasting out across the ward.

I was retaining fluid in a big way, so I was given (in the words of an oncologist, reading my file later) "a massive dose" of Lasix[36]. That had me standing in the corner, clutching a bottle, tapping my foot nervously, and thinking about designs for automatic watering systems.

As is usual when prescribing large doses of diuretics, fluid balance monitoring was set in place. In this instance, the job fell to a young nurse and an even younger student operating under her influence. They obviously hated one another and did not exchange a single word in my hearing over an eight hour shift. Nor did they ever speak to the patient.

---

[36] **Lasix** (*frusemide* or *furosemide*) is a diuretic that prevents your body from absorbing too much salt. This allows the salt to instead be passed in your urine. It is used to treat fluid retention in people with congestive heart failure, liver disease, or a kidney disorder such as nephrotic syndrome. Lasix is also used to treat high blood pressure (hypertension).

I watched them come, scowling, into my cubicle and fiddle about. The outgoing portion was simple to check; they took away the bottle, measured and recorded the contents and brought back a fresh container.

The tricky part was the intake measurement. On an overway table at the end of the bed was a yellow jug containing Adelaide tap water[37]. I grew up in a place where the water has no superfluous colour, flavour, or odour, so I don't drink Adelaide tap water. I had asked three times for the yellow jug to be removed. Each time it had been replaced by someone else, in satisfaction of a compulsion shared by most of the staff.

While in this ward, I was drinking iced tea provided in bottles by my wife. The nurses never asked, so they never learned this central fact. Instead, they would come into the cubicle and study the yellow jug. They would heft it, jiggle it, and eye the water level, which did not change over the course of their shift. What they wrote on the Fluid Balance Chart remains a mystery. You'd think someone would notice a zero intake and question the patient, but, no, that wasn't considered necessary here.

The next item of interest was the arrival of a nurse with two syringes in one hand. She had them splayed between her fingers and was waving them about like a costume element in a corroboree. Her attitude was that *This-Is-All-A-Game* and *Aren't-I-Cute!* I thought her a fool and potentially dangerous to patients.

Two Syringes said that one of them contained insulin; I forget what was in the other one. I administer my own insulin. I wouldn't trust her anywhere near me with a syringe and I told her so. This brought out the bully in her. She attempted to

---

[37] **Adelaide tap water** has a sorry history. For decades it was said that passing ships would take on water anywhere in the world, except Adelaide and Aden. Adelaide tap water used to have a charming brown tinge to it, but recent filtration improvements have removed that. Now the only concern is the taste. Some people swear that it has no taste, others (more sensitive souls) know better. The divide in opinion usually reflects the water one grew up drinking.

browbeat me into obedience. I told her I had no time for bullies and asked her to leave.

Ten minutes later she returned and opened with, "The compromise I'm prepared to accept is..."

I said, "There will be no compromise. Please go away."

Fifteen minutes later her boss turned up. While marginally more polite, she maintained the fiction that nurses are all-knowing and patients are required to submit on command. I asked her to leave.

The next visitor was a doctor. She spoke to me like a grown-up and listened when I spoke. I told her that insulin is a dangerous drug. I reminded her that we'd recently had the court case in Australia where a nurse was charged with murdering patients she didn't like with insulin they didn't need. I repeated that I administered my own insulin.

The doctor was smart enough not to get into a fight. She suggested that I administer the insulin, while a nurse observed and recorded the details.

No problem, I could do that.

Of course, Two Syringes was to be the observer. That was fine with me. I laid out the equipment on the bed and waited. Five minutes later, Two Syringes wandered into the cubicle, saw the insulin pen on the bed, and exclaimed "Ah, insulin!" She grabbed my file and read out loud as she wrote that she had observed me take so many units of insulin, then she flounced out.

I hadn't touched the pen, I hadn't taken any insulin, I was as in need as previously, but the paperwork showed me as having received a full dose.

I went into shock.

Five minutes later, Two Syringes came past. I asked her, "What just happened?"

She gave me a special *Aren't-I-Cute!* smile and said: "I was multitasking and needed to do some other things."

I asked, "Have you ever heard of *perjury*? Have you ever heard of the *Coroner's Court*? Have you ever heard of *prison*?"

She gave a dismissive smirk and wandered away. I thought about making a fuss, but I knew that if I did the offending document would disappear, be replaced by another, and I would look like a liar. Mostly I couldn't believe what I'd just witnessed.

Stupidity bothers me, and these incidents have stayed in mind ever since.

A few weeks later, I met with my cardiologist. He put me through a range of tests, then sat me down in his office, where he asked a lot of questions. Eventually, I asked him, "What does it mean that I had a heart attack?"

He said, "I'm not convinced you did."

Whoa!

I couldn't say how many people at the hospital claimed that I had. Most of them had charged into an explanation of how I didn't notice any symptoms by talking about diabetes and *neuropathy*[38] and how my loss of feeling would account for my not noticing. It was as though the most important thing for them was to look like an expert on diabetes, rather than focus on the heart attack.

---

[38] **Neuropathy** is a nerve condition that can lead to pain, numbness or tingling in one or more parts of the body. One of the most common causes is diabetes and I do have a loss of feeling in my feet and hands.

In the hospital, we took to calling it a "secret heart attack," because I didn't notice. Now it seems that it was really an *imaginary* heart attack, and I wasn't the person doing the imagining.

The one thing they had was a measure of *troponin* in the blood. I asked the cardiologist about that. He said that a single reading tells us close to nothing. For an indication of a heart attack, you would need to see several readings, followed by a sharp increase. *That* would constitute evidence.

I had been puzzled by their initial excitement over the "heart attack," followed a few days later by disinterest, as I discharged myself and they didn't want to see me again for almost two months. Perhaps a dawning realisation that they had misread this one fed into a desire to have it quietly go away.

The hospital cardiologist did a round, listening to patient summaries from interns, asking questions, and making comments. He was a little man with Little Man Attitude. If you were taller than him, if you said anything he didn't like, if he didn't like how you looked, he would ridicule you or play some practical joke on you. He didn't like me; I failed all his tests.

So, just for a laugh, he booked me in for an angiogram. This required fasting from midnight. I spent a miserable day waiting for the call, only to learn mid-afternoon that he'd placed me at number nine on a list that wouldn't get past number six that day.

In other words, it was all for nothing. A little in-joke. Ha ha ha.

The other thing that happened that day was my overhearing a loud farmer's conversation about a relative who was taken to hospital after a heart attack and given an angiogram, which dislodged a clot in his heart. The clot travelled to his brain and he suffered a massive stroke. Three days later he was dead.

Whoops.

You pays your money and you takes your chances.

The consensus view now was that he should have been placed on blood thinners long enough for the clot to dissolve before any angiogram. Either way, I was suddenly happy to put that procedure off for a while.

On the Thursday evening, I received a unit of blood over a four hour period. It normally happened over an hour and a half, but they were being careful.

The next day I was taken for an echocardiogram, followed by the second unit of blood. Four hours later, all promises (bar the angiogram) had been delivered. I couldn't think of a reason to be in hospital, so I went home.

Chapter Twenty-Two

"Shark-oh."

"What?"

"Shark-oh fracture of the left foot."

I had arrived at my podiatrist's office for a boring routine treatment, but Melanie seized upon the swelling in my left foot as something significant. Worse than that, as something to worry about.

It turns out that Monsieur Charcot[39] was a pioneering French neurologist who has a bunch of medical problems named after him. *Charcot arthropathy* is one of the most serious foot problems that diabetics face. When a diabetic fractures a bone in the foot, he or she may not realize it because of nerve damage (neuropathy).

With Charcot arthropathy, we're talking about bone disintegration. If I continued to walk on the injured foot, it could result in more severe fractures and dislocations, trauma which could deform the shape of the foot.

If you're wondering how bad it can get, take a look at some of the photos on the internet.

---

[39] **Jean-Martin Charcot** (1825–1893) was a French neurologist and professor of anatomical pathology. Known as "the founder of modern neurology," he was the first to describe multiple sclerosis and Charcot arthropathy. His name has been associated with at least 15 medical eponyms, including Charcot–Marie–Tooth disease and Charcot disease (better known as amyotrophic lateral sclerosis, motor neurone disease, or Lou Gehrig disease).

In the space of two weeks, I'd managed to not notice a (possible) heart attack and not notice a broken foot. It is difficult to learn that and not start to wonder what other bits might be falling apart.

Melanie decided that the best way (the quickest way, the cheapest way) to get the x-rays we needed was a trip to the Emergency Department of our local friendly hospital. On my way over there, I picked up some food to guard against the hypoglycaemia which seems to follow me about.

I spent an hour or so in the waiting room, admiring my fellow patients, while gnawing through a baguette filled with ham, cheese, tomato and a persistent lettuce, which stuck to my teeth.

I scratched away at the teeth as I went through blood tests, E.C.G., and an ultrasound of my thigh.

The young doctor with the ultrasound machine started by groping around my gronicles and the wobbly member. I was getting ready to help him focus by jabbing a friendly finger in his eye, when I noticed that his assistant was a pretty student doctor. He was giving her all the attention the situation would bear. The bruising to the wobbly member and the chimes ringing out from the gronicles were merely collateral damage. I put the friendly finger back in its holster.

He was able to tear himself away from the student doctor long enough to tell me that there were no clots in my thigh.

That left the question of my foot. He thought that feet were a matter for podiatrists and wanted to send me back to see the podiatrist who had sent me here to see him.

After a trying six hours in the Emergency Department, I wanted a foot x-ray. I explained to him that the suggestion of broken bones in the foot matched the kind of pain I'd been experiencing. I said that I couldn't play football like this and wept piteously.

He wanted to look good in front of the student, so he booked the foot x-ray. By the time I got back, he'd left, the student had left, and everyone I'd met had left. So I went home, too. I like it at home.

Melanie arranged a choice of moon boots[40] for me. I chose the cute short ones, which didn't compress my calf muscles.

A couple of days later, someone rang from the hospital and said they were organising a referral to the diabetic foot clinic. I would be contacted in writing. This wasn't good enough for Melanie. She made some calls and, in double-quick time, I was sitting in the Podiatry Outpatient Clinic, listening to Carla, a hospital podiatrist.

She explained that the broken bone was in the middle of my foot, that it was a stage one, Charcot-related fracture, and that these conditions can turn horrific. She started to tell me in graphic detail of the damage and suffering that lay in wait if I didn't take a few sensible steps. I had to beg her to stop.

I had gone to the meeting with Carla hoping to learn that I had a simple problem with a simple solution. Instead I found that I had a complex problem with no solution and years of complex management required to make the best of things.

The boot I had so proudly purchased failed the Carla Test and now sits, shame-faced, in the corner, with its hands folded in its lap, and its head bowed.

I was sent down to the second floor, where I hobbled to the end of a corridor barely a mile long, to Orthotics & Prosthetics, to be

---

[40] A **moonboot**, so called, is actually a controlled ankle motion walking boot, or CAM boot, also sometimes called a below knee walking boot. It is a device prescribed for the treatment and stabilization of severe sprains, fractures, and tendon or ligament tears in the ankle or foot. In situations where ankle motion but not weight is to be limited, it may be used in place of a cast.

fitted with a larger boot. This turned out to be more supportive and comfortable than the other. Over the next week and a half, a shoe was built up to match the height of the boot.

The following week, I presented myself before the Multi-Disciplinary High Risk Foot Clinic. This august body had been given a big build-up, with everyone expressing high expectations. I was warned to be on time for the 9:00am appointment.

A sleepless night prepared me for the early arrival, but not for the long wait. They were well over an hour late.

I was escorted to a small room by Cathy Chatter, a middle-aged talking machine, who claimed to be a podiatrist. She told me to remove my boot/shoe and sit in the high chair, then she departed.

By the time she returned, I was seated, awkwardly, in the forward-leaning high chair. She pushed some buttons and I was tilted backwards, then raised toward the ceiling, like an offering to the gods on the subcontinent. I was expecting small birds to descend and peck at my eyes.

Miss Chatter continued her Wall-of-Sound impersonation. In among the flooding crowd of verbs and nouns, I recognised the statement that they couldn't find my file. She wondered aloud if I had another appointment at the hospital that day.

Before I could mention the fact that I'd been in the Oncology Day Centre for a transfusion a couple of days ago, she decided that anything I might say was obviously irrelevant, broke back into babble, and departed.

Again.

For about three quarters of an hour.

After fifteen minutes, the position I was trapped in had become so uncomfortable I needed to escape. A vertigo-inducing descent over the side followed, with a short hang time, then drop to the floor. A nasty exercise for someone like me in bare feet.

I sat for another thirty minutes in a normal chair, untroubled by human company.

The bare concrete floor under my bare feet grew ever colder. In desperation, I liberated a couple of brown paper bags from a cupboard and, hobo-like, employed them as foot warmers.

I was thinking of lighting a small fire when Cathy Chatter returned, lowered the high chair again, and ordered me back into it. I was being re-elevated when some other people entered the room through the back door. One of them said he was a vascular surgeon, a Dr. Pfhgumbumble or something.

I said, "Sorry, what was the name?"

The question angered him and he snarled a sharper version of "Dr. Pfhgumbumble." I never really got past the first three letters.

There was no encouragement for me to ask questions, so I shut up. Two other people were present. They didn't speak to me. No one offered their names. Perhaps they didn't have names. I was tempted to try "B1" or "B2", just to see what would happen, but my nerve failed.

There was a short conversation among the Nameless and Pfhgumbumble, then they departed through the front door. I thought, maybe they were going for refreshments. Cathy Chatter broke back into full power babble. I didn't know if she was filling the gap until the morning tea came in, or if she was feeding her compulsion.

With the benefit of hindsight, I think she was attempting a summary of options and a description of the likely path ahead.

I was permitted to return to earth and to replace my footwear. The Wall-of-Sound power babble continued a long time. I recognised references to two hospitals, to casts, singular and serial, and to O&P. These were sometimes Orthotics and Prosthetics, sometimes Orthopaedics and Prosthetics, but never Obstetrics and Prosthetics.

I finally tired of the endless sound and said, "Please stop talking."

This caused some offence, but even more shock. The one held the other in tension long enough for me to say that I had understood less than half of what she had said, and mentioned, in sequence, the two hospitals, casts, singular and serial, and O&P.

This triggered a fresh, but more focused, bout of verbal diarrhoea. O&P operate at both hospitals, so they can set and remove casts, willy-nilly, as required.

My assumption was that she had plaster casts in view, but I was never permitted to ask that question.

A cast can be singular or serial because they are the same thing, as any idiot knows. That's why they have two names. And there are two hospitals involved so that Orthopaedics can play a hand in all that is to follow.

Somewhere in the midst of this came a description of the Charcot foot phenomenon and treatment plan. Miss Chatter stated that there were three stages. I interjected that Carla thought there were five stages[41].

---

[41] My mistake. There are three stages:
Acute Stage – There is redness, swelling, and warmth in the foot. This can last for several weeks, during which dislocation and fragmentation of the bones may occur.
Subacute Stage – The damaged bones begin to come together. There is a reduction in the redness, swelling and warmth of the foot.
Chronic Stage – Reconstruction and consolidation. There is no longer any redness, swelling, or warmth. The bones have "healed" (read *hardened*), but they are typically deformed from their original appearance.

That did not go down well. Chatter dismissed the validity of all understanding other than her own, then continued in a higher key.

All I understood of what followed related to a speculative consideration of the distant future. I was desperately trying to understand my next move, or maybe two. The longer term could await its time.

Miss Chatter became agitated about the need for some orchestration in the timetables of O&P and Carla, the podiatrist, so that Carla could be present when the cast was not. She decided that my phone number had taken on sudden significance and left the room.

I sat quietly and waited.

Miss Chatter returned, recited my number, asked if that was correct and, on my affirmation, departed again.

I sat quietly and waited.

After another fifteen minutes, a young woman walked into the room and demanded to know who I was and what I was doing there. I surrendered my name; that seemed sufficient.

The young woman became agitated and told me I had been dismissed; the session was over; there was no more to add; no further questions would be answered; the game had passed me by; I had achieved obsolescence, and was now surplus to requirement.

I mumbled something about the show being a shambles and started to walk out. This seemed to worry the young woman and she asked when my next appointment was with Carla. I told her there wasn't one and kept walking.

The young woman darted into a side room, emerged and ran after me, shouting that someone would send me a letter[42].

I got into the lift and left.

---

[42] No such letter was ever received and I never saw Carla or Cathy Chatter again.

Chapter Twenty-Three

I attended what should have been a routine three-monthly appointment with Dr. Tease, only to learn that he was no longer about the place. He had folded his tent and melted into the night.

More accurately, he had been placed on "unexpected long-term leave," the circumstances surrounding which were subject to a gag order. It was all very mysterious. In the ultimate tease, he was no longer available for discussion. Eleven years of personal association evaporated in a heart-beat.

In the wash up from the Multi-Disciplinary High Risk Foot debacle, I attended the Outpatients Clinic at Hospital Two to meet with an orthopaedic surgeon. My wife and I arrived by bus at stop 21 in the firm belief that we would be outside the hospital. And we were. About two kilometres outside.

So we trudged, and we plodded, and we slogged, and we dragged ourselves slowly through the undergrowth of the maze that encompasses the cunningly hidden entrance, until at last we were inside the hospital, where we fell upon the nearest comfort station in vocal celebration of the opportunity afforded for personal relief.

Sometime later, I made my way to the nearest Information booth, where an earnest woman gave directions to Area 2, which was located conveniently on the opposite side of the hospital.

By then, my wife had emerged, given a final celebratory cry of relief, and she joined me on the long trek to the far side, only to discover that we were in the wrong place. We needed Area 3, which lies somewhere in the middle.

After a bout of preliminary paper work, and thirty minutes of rest in the waiting area, I was inducted into a small room, where I removed all footwear.

The removal of my shoe revealed that the dressing that Melanie, my podiatrist, had so carefully placed on the big toe of my non-Charcot foot the day previous was now askew, worn ragged and blood-stained. People gathered to stare. Questions were asked. Notes were taken. While under heavy interrogation, I might have let slip her name as the author of the dressing. I'm ashamed to have to report that.

The orthopaedic surgeon was a crusty old woman who felt herself to be much put upon. Apparently the Multi-Disciplinary High Risk Foot thing was supposed to be a Hospital One show, with Dr. Crusty merely acting as a consultant, but all the diabetes-related foot problems were being dumped on her. For example, she received three new Charcot cases[43] in the week when I was first mentioned.

Charcot foot cases are unpopular within much of the medical profession. This has something to do with the historical fact the disease was first reported in France in 1883 (the year Coco Chanel was born and the French conquered Viet Nam) and most early cases involved people who had syphilis.

Syphilis is rare in Australia today, with diabetes having taken up the slack. Nonetheless the prejudice perseveres that Charcot foot cases are all degenerates, debt collectors or drunkards. I have to confess to having had a youthful fling with debt collecting, but it's in the distant past now. The twelve-step program helped me a great deal.

---

[43] Charcot foot cases are rare. Neither my G.P. of over twenty years nor my podiatrist of over fifteen years has seen another in private practice.

The bloody toe saga erupted after a shoe was built up to match the height of the moon boot and thus reduce stress on my hips. The shoe sloped forward, to aid in walking, but had the side effect of pressing the toes into the end of the shoe. The morning's peregrinations had shaved another layer of skin from the big toe.

Dr. Crusty described the problem to her team at great length until, finally, the Orthotics and Prosthetics (O&P) guy, leaping into action, seized the shoe and headed for his laboratory.

In his absence, the dressing on my toe was removed and replaced. The O&P Guy returned with shoe in hand. He had stretched out the toe and was keen to learn if this would solve the problem. He applied a bright red lipstick (from his personal collection) to the new dressing on the big toe and inserted a white paper lining inside the shoe. I was reshoed, like a favourite racehorse, and sent off for an x-ray (on the other foot).

On my return, red lipstick was found to be smeared all over the paper lining. The shoe was rejected as unsuitable and I was issued with a cute Japanese-style healing shoe.

All talk about plaster casts was placed on hold. I retained the moon boot, along with a supplement of yellow crutches.

The phrase of the day was "non-weight bearing." The foot had to be allowed to reach stage two without further damage being inflicted, if we hoped to achieve a "shoe-able" foot in the long term. To this end, I had to absolutely stay off that foot.

Of course, I didn't. It's too hard to live your life while never taking a step or two in pursuit of something you need.

I did poorly with the crutches, as the arthritis had robbed me of hand strength. My reward for a disappointing foot x-ray a month later was to have my foot encased in a total contact cast[44]. For a week. Then the plaster cast was removed.

The idea of a cast didn't bother me, not once I'd experienced the moonboot for a while. It was the idea of having the cast *cut off* that made me nervous.

A white-haired man opened a cupboard filled with angle grinders of various sizes. He selected one, hefted it, while deciding if he liked it enough to use it on me, then launched into his task with enthusiasm.

He cut the outline of a lid from the top of the cast, then attacked the next layer with two-handed levering tools and industrial scissors. The lid surrendered to the onslaught and was tossed aside. My leg was lifted out and the rest of the cast joined the lid in the bin. I was free. My leg was dirty, sweaty, and covered in powdered plaster, but free of the weight of the cast.

My wife, who'd been watching with interest, brought out her all-purpose scissors and trimmed my toenails. A nurse came and washed the leg. Ah, bliss.

The only downside was the emaciated look of the calf. Shrunken, wrinkled, flabby. Ugly. The price of immobilising my leg.

A foot x-ray followed, then another orthopaedic surgeon showed me the pictures on a computer. The reality looked so much better than the scene of devastation I'd been imagining.

Over the weeks that followed, a routine developed whereby, every Monday, the cast was cut off, the foot admired, then x-rayed, and a new cast moulded in place.

---

[44] A **total contact cast** (TCC) is designed to reduce pressure on an injury. It involves encasing the toes, foot and lower leg in a plaster cast. This redistributes pressure from the foot into the leg during everyday movements, allowing the injury to heal.

Finally, Dr. Crusty decided that things had progressed so well, I could move to a CROW[45] boot. Measurements were taken. A special cast was formed around my leg, cut down the middle, then levered apart while I wriggled my leg free. This would be the model for the CROW boot to come.

In the meantime, my biggest problem was keeping myself clean. A shower was a problematic exercise, as a wet cast is a weak cast. On the first Monday that I was booked in for cast removal, I worried that half a bottle of aftershave wouldn't be enough to disguise the pong[46] I was producing.

I raided my stash of plastic shopping bags, selected several large ones with the names of designer labels on them, erected a shelter around the plaster cast, using bags and sticky tape in a method modelled on the wattle-and-daub style of house construction favoured by the early settlers; then I braved the shower.

My structure leaked.

Not badly, but enough so that everyone at the hospital noticed. Loud enquiries were made. Opinions were expressed. There was surprise, shock, disappointment. Muttered comments were made concerning the state of my mental health. The water / plaster problem was explained to me in several tones of voice and with a conscious effort to reduce the concept to the level a child could understand. A really stupid child.

It was a humiliating day at the office.

---

[45] CROW: **Charcot Restraint Orthotic Walker**; a stable boot designed to accommodate and support a foot with Charcot neuroarthropathy. It is custom-made for each patient. The outer shell consists of two plastic or fiberglass clamshell pieces that are strapped together with Velcro. It is sturdy and can prevent other bones from cracking or breaking. The bottom of the boot has a rounded rocker-bottom shape, and can be walked on. The boot contains a custom, removable foam insole, which provides even support to the entire foot.
[46] **Pong**: British slang for odour, especially an unpleasant odour.

Some time in the next week, my wife went on a medical supplies safari and turned up several boxes of *Waterproof Leg Protectors*[47] and a fresh supply of duct tape. Applied properly, the duct tape sealed the top of the Leg Protectors, keeping everything inside dry, then assisted with hair removal following the shower.

But if the Protectors did a great job of keeping water out, they did an even better job of keeping water in, once a leak had been sprung. Or so I discovered during my final shower under plastic. I looked down in the midst of a joyful burst of soaping, scrubbing and rinsing, only to see that my plasterised foot was inside an improvised swimming pool, its head under water, and going down for the third time.

There followed a panic-stricken snipping of the bag, a rush of water as the foot was lifted out, some superficial towelling, and a sloshing walk to the chair, where I sat while a hair dryer was applied. This produced a dry exterior of all the cast, except the heel, the lowest point in my reclining check mark of a leg.

The heel leaked. Constantly. Annoyingly. Embarrassingly. All night long. I kept it wrapped in a towel, which localised the damp spot, but did nothing to cure the problem.

We travelled to the hospital next morning, where I braced for a chiding[48]. I had rehearsed a story which involved me in a journey to the highest room in the tallest tower to rescue a princess, only to fall into the deepest hole in the darkest forest, and find myself swimming for my life, while beating off leeches, flesh-eating crabs and tiger snakes. At two in the morning, the story seemed reasonable. By daylight, I had doubts.

---

[47] Made by *Surgipack* in Guangdong, China.
[48] Yes, a *chiding*. To chide is to admonish, berate, castigate, chastise, rebuke, reprimand, reproach, reprove, scold, upbraid. In *Die Hard With a Vengeance* (1995), Jeremy Irons said he was going to send Samuel L. Jackson home "with a chiding," but changed his mind.

The O&P guy didn't buy it. He wanted the truth; which, once furnished, proved a lot less interesting than my original offering.

The cast remained just as wet. It was quickly removed, the leg was washed, and a knee-high white sock fitted. Then a black CROW boot came out and I suddenly looked like I was ready for a *KISS* tribute concert. I just needed more makeup, a second boot, and a longer tongue.

My leg was emaciated, ugly. My foot, uglier. The toenails frightening. We rang Melanie and were rewarded with an afternoon appointment at the podiatrist's, where extensive snipping removed a pile of debris and left a recognisable foot. Promises were made that the rest would recover in time.

So here I was, stage two Charcot foot, shrivelled leg, well-clipped toenails, a shiny black CROW boot in place, and less than a year to go in terms of achieving our ultimate goal: one "shoe-able" foot. I had high hopes[49].

---

[49] The time frame in this book is flexible. This event took place in August; the next chapter occurred in June. One problem at a time...

Chapter Twenty-Four

On the Queen's Birthday[50] Monday, I had a transfusion in the morning. I was eager to get home to watch a football match on television, and encouraged staff to hurry it up a bit. That evening I had a reaction (for the first time ever) and developed acute congestive cardiac failure (C.C.F.) with arrhythmia. It was not a pleasant experience.

We rang for an ambulance about 8:30pm. I thought the problem was asthma-related, due to the uncontrolled rapid breathing. The ambos placed me on oxygen and encouraged me to take deep breaths. And I would have, if I could have, but my lungs were almost full of fluid.

They proceeded to lay me back in the ambulance chair and strap me in. This was the worst possible position for someone with acute C.C.F. I struggled to free myself and sit up, but they fought me, until I decided that the fastest way out of this was to go through the journey and get out at the other end, if I was still alive. I felt close to death and people who saw me at the Emergency Department made comments to that effect in the days that followed.

Once inside the Emergency Department, I sat up with my feet over the side and continued to breathe in rapid shallow breaths. I remained in that basic posture, in different locations, for the next two days.

---

[50] The tradition of an annual celebration of the British sovereign's birthday began in 1748. The date of the event varies. In South Australia it falls on the second Monday in June. In Australia, the event involves a public holiday, the presentation of the Queen's Birthday Honours List and the playing of a football match between the Collingwood and Melbourne Football Clubs.

In the Emergency Department, I had a chest x-ray, an E.C.G. and sundry other tests. The expression I heard used most was "A.P.O." (acute pulmonary oedema[51] [52]).

Then I was moved to the High Dependency Intensive Care Unit. This was a large room, with heavy curtaining, my own fulltime nurse and a part-time doctor. The nurse was new at this and eager to learn. The doctor was new at this and eager to practice. On me.

I was loaded up with needles, like a pin cushion. There was an arterial line, two cannulas (*two*, just in case), with more failed attempts at finding a useful vein than successful, plus ECG wires, a pulse oximeter[53] and a blood pressure cuff. I was injected with a bunch of drugs, primarily diuretic and cardiac medications.

Then I was placed in a CPAP (Continuous Positive Airways Pressure) mask. This is a device invented by Darth Vader in an act of revenge. A CPAP seals around your mouth and nose. It is fixed tightly in position, then oxygen is pumped in in a controlled manner, in an attempt to force you to breathe the way they want you to.

When this first happened to me, the sensation was beyond weird. When I wanted to breathe in, the machine was breathing out and I got nothing. Then the machine forced a huge amount of air into my lungs, no matter that I was wanting to breathe out. Then there were moments when the air was neither coming nor going, and I felt as though I had been dropped into a vacuum.

---

[51] **Acute pulmonary oedema** is fluid accumulation in the tissue and air spaces of the lungs. It leads to impaired gas exchange and can result in fatal respiratory distress or cardiac arrest.

[52] **"Oedema"** is the original British/Australasian spelling, taken from the Greek word *oídēma* meaning "swelling". The American version drops the 'o' in the interests of simplicity and efficiency. Australians are stuck with the British version on account of the convicts, and all that.

[53] **Pulse oximeters** are small, lightweight monitors that attach to a fingertip. They use light to measure the oxygen level (oxygen saturation) of the blood.

The early stages were frightening, but things settled down as Darth and I learned to waltz together.

Over the time, I was placed in three masks of different design. The first, and largest, enclosed my eyes as well as mouth and nose. This was a hassle because I was sweating like a porcine beast. The sweat ran into my eyes and there was nothing I could do about it.

The big mask was also the noisiest. When you hear Darth Vader (from the outside), his breathing has a nice regular sound to it. When you hear it from inside the mask, it sounds like a small Cessna trying to take off.

That, mixed with the sound of my sobbing, made it hard to hear the doctor, especially when she told me that I probably agreed with her idea to insert a catheter[54].

I probably didn't agree and yelled that I rated her idea "F.I.". She took this to involve some form of expletive-based abuse. I hurried to explain that this was the Final Insult. They'd been everywhere else I never wanted anyone to go. All that was left was an assault on the wobbly member, and here we were.

So, at three o'clock on a Tuesday morning, two attractive young women stripped me naked from the waist down. Then they went to work, or more accurately, the doctor went to work on me.

In Australia, a nurse can install a catheter on a woman, but not on a man. That's in the purview of doctors only, due to the higher degree of difficulty.

---

[54] **Catheters** are medical devices that can be inserted into a body cavity, duct, or vessel in the body to allow drainage, administration of fluids or gases, access by surgical instruments, or other tasks. Catheters can be tailored for cardiovascular, urological, gastrointestinal, neurovascular, and ophthalmic applications.

The nurse mostly helped by gathering up belly flab by the armful and holding it out of the way. She had a cute way of saying, "I'm going to touch your face" (to adjust the mask), "I'm going to touch your tummy," and so on. The doctor never said, "I'm going to grab you by the cock," but that's what happened.

She applied a liberal dose of some liquid to the member and gave the unit a thorough rub in an attempt to remove the outer layer of sweat and germs.

In the days of my youth, this would have resulted in the wobbly member leaping to his feet and looking about in search of romance and adventure, but on this cold winter's night, I had nothing. Not a flicker, not a twitch, not even a tremble.

I was still more wrestling with Darth than waltzing at the time, and preoccupied with trying to avoid the periods of vacuum breath, so I only barely heard the doctor say, "I'm going to apply some local anaesthetic. It might hurt a bit going in."

It might hurt a bit. Make a note of that.

I'd like to point out that I was now six hours into this hospital visit and had been the target of numerous needle assaults on my body. I didn't complain once. The nurse commented on this; the doctor commented on this. Meek as a lamb. Taking the rough with the smooth, and never a murmur.

Then she forced something inside the wobbly member in a manner contrary to all natural process. A place where liquids come out had a rusted iron pipe forced in. My body convulsed with pain and I bellowed, "FAAARK THAT HURTS!"

The pain subsided slowly, but a bond had been broken. When the doctor later asked if we were still friends, the best I could do was say, "I'm thinking about it."

And so things muddled along. They experimented with different masks, different rates of oxygen flow. Shifts came and went. I didn't eat, I didn't drink, I didn't take my medications. I especially didn't take any insulin. In my brief moments of clarity, I worried about the insulin.

A cardiologist from the Outpatients Cardiology Unit came to see me. His advice boiled down to this: The Public and Private systems don't mix. You end up with too many cooks. He thought I should stick with my cardiologist and do wherever he wanted me to do. That seemed to make sense.

At every shift change, a bunch of doctors gathered at the door and someone gave an account of the exhibit on display.

At the time, I was seated in a darkened room. On my left hand, I had an arterial line, two cannulas, and a pulse oximeter. The pulse oximeter had a red light at the end. When I extended my hand, it looked like the glowing finger of E.T. from *E.T. the Extra-Terrestrial*.

At one shift change, as the doctors took up their viewing positions, I slowly raised my left hand. This mesmerised them, and they all stared. I waited a long beat, then said, in a clearly enunciated monotone: "I Come In Peace For All Mankind."

It remains a proud fact that two doctors laughed out loud. It's tough to get a doctor to laugh out loud. The dude running the show said, "Mister Sheppard is feeling well in himself." Which I was. I was alive, something that had seemed unlikely on the Monday.

Late that night I requested assistance to get out of a chair that had been brought in as an experiment. I hated that chair; it trapped me like a wild animal. The nurse asked me what I would do if I got out.

To explain: I was coated with many hours' worth of the kind of sweat which is only secreted during cardiac distress. I had been folded into the same basic position for many, many hours and my flesh had begun to adhere to itself. My gronicles stuck to my thigh, alongside the duct tape which held the rusted iron pipe in place. If I moved, one piece of flesh tore away from another piece of flesh.

It was painful. It was embarrassing. I had no underwear on, so my shame was on permanent display to the neighbourhood.

I had begun to dream of a hot shower the way a hungry man dreamed of steak and chips. The thought of a handful of talcum powder splashed about the area made me go weak at the knees.

So, when asked what I would do, I answered in three words which—to my mind—drew all these strands into a single coherent thought. I would, I said, scratch my balls.

Now it turns out that men are only allowed to employ the word "balls" in a sentence if they have gained approval from the local Political Correctness Committee, in writing, and well in advance. I had failed that test.

And, as the only kind of people who would employ "balls" in a sentence, unapproved, were the criminally insane, I was to be regarded as an object of derision.

There followed a long harangue consisting of feminist slogans, which if only I had memorised them, would have made me a better person.

For the first time since I landed in the Emergency Department, I felt unsafe. This angry ranting woman had access to endless drugs and sharp metallic objects. She frightened me. I'm not worried by lesbians, but gangs of angry young women are dangerous. Three of such levered me out of the chair and dragged it out of the room, leaving me only echoes of militant slogans for company.

I spent several hours considering my position. I no longer needed the Darth Vader mask. I was receiving no ongoing physical therapy. Any medication I was taking here, I could take at home. In short, I couldn't think of a single reason to stay, so I decided to go home.

Chapter Twenty-Five

"I'm going home," I said.

This is known in the trade as a "Discharge Against Medical Advice."

It's a practice that doctors hate. They want the control, the final say. With the good ones, it reflects their genuine hope for your best outcome. With the others, well...

The problem I find with even the best-intentioned doctors is that they have a narrow focus. They find it difficult to step back and see the bigger, more human perspective.

The first piece of Medical Advice I ever received came when I was twenty-two years old. A prominent surgeon had operated to remove a lump from my left axilla[55] and, afterwards, announced that I would be dead[56] before I was twenty-five.

At the time of writing this, I am sixty-three. I conclude that not all medical advice is to be blindly trusted. Had I listened to that doctor, I would have laid down and died, and missed out on decades of drama, romance and adventure, love and laughter, plus large slabs of really boring stuff. And a fair bit of misery. But you get the idea.

It upset a lot of people when I announced that I was going home. They formed a queue and took turns at telling me why I had to

---

[55] This is a complicated area to define, but for our purposes, it refers to the underarm, i.e., the hollow beneath the junction of the arm and shoulder.
[56] *Did a doctor really say you'd "be dead" within three years?* Yes, he did, but he was speaking over the phone to a theatre sister (an OR nurse) with whom he had worked for years, not thinking that she was also a young wife.

stay. The most emotional of these was the author of the Final Insult. She was taking it personally and her feelings were reflected in her angry tone. I had to ask her to lower her voice.

She thought I needed to stay to see someone from the Cardiology team. I explained that I'd already had a good session with a hospital cardiologist and that he had suggested I stick with my private practice cardiologist. Too many cooks and all that.

She admitted that that was good advice and, from that point, her arguments fell apart, but her emotional commitment to keeping me in the system did not soften. She was called away to see another patient and we never got to complete our discussion.

The other major expression of concern came from a senior clinician. He said they had just started me on a course of antibiotics and wanted me to stay so they could monitor my progress and, if necessary, tweak the dosage.

I had been on daily antibiotics for a year at a time, in conjunction with the chemotherapy, so wasn't worried about minor fiddling that might make sense in a perfect world, but seemed a bit much in the rough and tumble of a life lived with leukaemia.

He wanted — with my permission — to talk to my private practice cardiologist about the situation. That intrigued me. I was supposed to see him in a day or so, anyway, as a follow-up to the question of whether or not I'd had a "secret" heart attack, so any interaction would be welcome.

He made the call, talked a long time, then handed the phone to me. Dr. Heart said he'd like to transfer me to a private hospital, partly so he could monitor my progress, but mostly so he could get a haematologist involved: the frequency of my blood transfusions had been increasing for some time and no one knew why. It might be time to organise my favourite tests, a CT scan and a bone marrow biopsy.

I agreed.

Hospital Three has a major cardiac focus. I was transferred by ambulance to their Acute Cardiac Unit and set up in a shared room with another bloke. I fell asleep and woke six hours later, a minor record for me. There was no chance I'd be getting back to sleep soon, so I chatted with the night nurse. She decided this was as good a time as any to remove the catheter.

A look of terror crossed my face.

"What," she asked, "have you got to worry about?"

"The blood, the pain, the screaming."

She gave a snort, one that signified a degree of intolerance for the spineless elements of society, then, in a few economical motions, had the paraphernalia deflated, disconnected, and packed away.

I didn't feel the rusted iron tube depart and needed to grope myself, slowly and carefully, to be sure it was gone. Earlier, if I so much as bumped something in the region, a sharp shock would pulse through the collection and fresh blood appeared in the urine bag. Now I could reposition the full set, both the hairy and the smooth, wrap it all gently in a surplus piece of cotton gown, and fall back in the bed with a huge sigh of relief.

All I needed was a shower.

Morning broke slowly in this part of the world. My roommate was going home, so he was up early, showered and dressed. I waited a decent interval, then headed for the bathroom. This represented an architect's creative use of waste space: a wide, flat triangle, with the hand bowl in one corner, the toilet in the opposite corner, as far away as possible, and the shower at the top.

I sat on the toilet and organised my towel, toiletries and change of clothes. There was a solid hand rail next to me and another at the back of the shower, and nothing anywhere else. I had to hobble on a broken foot across the cold, wet hinterland to the security of the shower handrail. Once there I hurried to turn on the hot tap. As that warmed up, I reached for the cold tap to adjust the temperature, but there was no cold tap.

There was no cold tap!

Seriously.

I hunted high, I hunted low. There was a hot tap, but no cold tap.

The water coming out of the shower nozzle was now scaldingly hot. The room filled with steam. I turned the water off, then hobbled to the door and asked my roommate, who was dressed and about to walk out the door, where was the cold tap?

He laughed and laughed. At the time, I thought he was laughing at the stupidity of a private hospital that couldn't afford the price of a dedicated cold tap. Later, I wondered if he were really laughing at his own private joke on me.

The one thing he did do was confirm that there was no cold tap; I wasn't hallucinating. That's always nice to know.

A nurse came in to tidy the room after Laughing Man's departure. She confirmed that there was no cold tap.

"The temperature is pre-set," she said.

Pre-set? What does that mean?

Was I supposed to fill out a form on admission, where I indicated my shower temperature preference and have someone at the front desk jiggle the controls for me? What if I wanted a cold shower?

I was laughing in disbelief. This was my first time in this expensive private hospital. Call me a peasant, but I like to adjust my shower water down to a tolerable level. I'd been waiting days for this shower. I had dreamed of taking this shower. And now I had to choose between boiling water or no water.

I sat on the toilet and thought about things. Maybe if I sprayed the shower water high into the air and allowed it to fall like rain, maybe it would cool down enough to become bearable. I had to find out.

The first few seconds of bathroom rain were tolerable, but then everything warmed up and I feared I was going to injure myself. I turned the water off.

The experiment had done enough to freshen up the sweat, but not enough to remove any of it. I sat on the toilet and towelled myself vigorously, thus removing one layer. The rest would have to wait until I got home, where we had a shower with two taps, one hot and one cold.

I hobbled back to the bed. Another nurse arrived. The day shift. I invited her to try the shower temperature. She stuck her hand under the water, quickly withdrew it, then announced that she would get the engineer to come and fix things. Tomorrow the shower would be fine.

The engineer?

I was still laughing in disbelief. No engineer had ever set foot in my bathroom at home, yet we adjusted the shower temperature daily. No problem: we had a cold tap.

I later learned that there was a regulator in the bathroom, which could alter the temperature of the hot water. When I was relocated to a single room that afternoon, I went searching for it, and — sure enough — there it was, high on the wall, almost out of reach. I experimented until I found a comfortable temperature, then had a long, soapy shower. The sweat came off and I felt clean all over.

Dr. Heart came by. He said that a haematologist would visit me later. This proved to be a tall, large man of Indian origin, who compensated for his impressive size by speaking softly. He indicated that he needed to conduct some tests. The first were a collection of different blood tests. It took the needle jockey a long time and a couple of attempts to find veins that would surrender enough blood.

No sooner was the blood taken, than word came down that Dr. Softly had arranged for me to have a CT scan that evening. I needed to start fasting for it right away.

A few hours later, I was collected by an orderly who carted me off to the radiology area, where I eventually found myself back on the Pizza Hut tray, propped in place by a stack of vinyl pillows. The young radiographer, who had a habit of saying things like, "Just a couple of seconds," then disappearing for fifteen minutes, took charge. He had me flat on my back for at least thirty minutes before finally announcing that he was ready to begin.

"Feeling happy, are we?"

"I'd rather feel safe, than happy."

"Okay, then. Just lining things up..."

I couldn't see any of what was happening and contented myself with coughing the C.C.F. cough that had been freshened up by this long stint spent flat on my back. The tray started to move, then my foot — my right foot, not the broken foot — smacked into the side of the big white donut.

I bellowed, mostly out of fear of what else this idiot had prepared for me. He was apologetic, shuffled the pillows, and tried again.

We made multiple passes through the eye of the needle, with him instructing me not to breathe, then not to cough, then to breathe but not cough. I managed the third alternative okay and we were done. Another orderly whisked me back to my room.

It was now about seven thirty at night. I got dressed in civilian attire, then wandered down to the nurses' station in search of dinner. There wasn't any. When you're fasting, your meals vanish. But they found a couple of stale sandwiches I could have. Lucky me.

I asked where the nearest exit was, as I was going to Hungry Jack's, a fast food joint a couple of hundred yards away, to get something to eat. This caused consternation. An acute cardiac unit patient roaming the streets, in the dark, with a broken foot in a moonboot? OMG! It was unheard of! It was unimaginable! It was positively indecent!

The resulting gab-fest took a few minutes to resolve. I thanked them for their concern, but I thought it reasonable that I be allowed an evening meal. There were a few half-hearted attempts at compromise, but I ended up taking the long walk to the main door and out into the cold, dark night.

I know it sounds silly, but this little rebellion of mine was a kind of celebration of life. And a way of shaking off the missing cold tap and the hassles with the CT scan. This was me being a kid celebrating the end of school year. Or something.

My wife and I used to eat at this fast food joint forty years earlier, so there was a small romantic element to the visit as well.

I didn't expect the night to be as cold, or the road noise to be quite that loud, or the walk to be so far, or the food to be that bad. I sat and ate and talked to my wife on the phone. Once she fully grasped where I was, I got the frosty reception I probably deserved. I sat longer than I might have, as the walk had taken more out of me than I expected.

Getting old is something that sneaks up on you from behind, and suddenly slaps you across the side of the head for no particular reason. There is no known defence; you just have to put up with it.

I was halfway back across the major arterial road, waiting for the lights to change, when I checked my phone. Three missed calls, all from the hospital. I had people worried. The lights changed; I shuffled on. As I reached the other side, I recognised a small figure, one of the nurses, come to rescue me. She escorted me back the short way, via the emergency entrance.

The next day, various ones shared a wink or a sly smile. Most of them had been cheering for me to succeed. One confessed she had been hoping I'd come back with a box of chocolates. It was something I'd thought of, but Hungry Jack's don't run to chocolates and no other store had been open.

I was booked in for a bone marrow biopsy four days later, on the following Monday. That left a lot of hanging about time, a lot of waiting.

The highlight was the student nurse who woke me up out of a deep sleep to ask if there was anything he could do for me. All I could think of was the wet towels on the bathroom floor. Could he take those out and bring some clean ones?

He didn't say "yes," he didn't say "no;" instead he started to interrogate me. Had I had a shower? At what time had I had that shower? Who advised me to have that shower?

It seems he was yet another tribal chief's son, who was above picking up wet towels, as he thought he should be running the hospital. I asked him to leave and not come back.

There was no laundry basket anywhere within sight, otherwise I'd have removed the towels myself. Instead, I learned to dump them on the floor in the doorway, within sight of every passer-by. The wet towels would vanish and be replaced by clean ones, with no interrogation necessary.

I dozed a lot, and was dozing still when they came for me. I woke in Recovery, passed their little tests, like wriggling my fingers and toes, and was whisked back to my room, where another male nurse was waiting for me. He launched into a bombastic speech in which he outlined the tablets I'd failed to take earlier. He was here to correct my failures, and thrust a plastic cup full of pills and a glass of water at me. I closed my eyes and feigned sleep.

Eventually he left.

My biggest concern was the steadily falling haemoglobin. One thing about being an in-patient was the daily blood test, which allowed me to monitor my decline. I'd dipped below the trigger point for a blood transfusion several days earlier and had only hung around Hospital Three for the bone marrow biopsy. Now that was done, I needed to get out and plug back into the Oncology Day Centre system.

I'd tried to discuss the problem with Dr. Heart and with Dr. Softly and with most of the nurses who'd walked into my room. No one wanted to engage with the question. They all fobbed me off with some reference to the bone marrow biopsy, as if that had something to do with my falling haemoglobin.

Doubtless, there was a mechanism for obtaining the needed blood transfusion at Hospital Three; it's just that I didn't know what that was, or how I could trigger the process. If I wanted to stay alive, I had to get out.

I had a cannula in the inside of my right forearm; a terrible position as it caught on everything. The sides of the bed were all up, trapping me as in a cage.

Then the Tablet Man walked back in. He repeated his tablet speech and thrust a plastic cup full of pills and a glass of water at me.

This was my sixth day in this hospital. I'd lost count of how many nurses I'd told that I can't take tablets with water; I can only take them with food. The fact should be plastered all over my file. It was obvious Tablet Man hadn't bothered to read the file.

I asked him how much he knew about me, about my medical condition. His first response was to bullshit me.

"Oh, I know lots about you." Then he changed the subject.

I tried again. "Tell me what you know about me, what you know about my medical condition."

His second response was to get angry. "I know your name, that you're in this ward and that I'm looking after you. That's enough." Then he stormed out of the room.

He later returned, having decided he needed to at least look like he was working with his patient.

I asked him to remove the cannula. He refused. I asked him to lower the side of the bed. He refused. Instead he launched into a lecture about how we had to work together. I cut him off and told him I wasn't interested. He seemed genuinely surprised, and asked why not.

"You're lazy. Too lazy to read my file. Too lazy to ask me any questions. Too lazy to listen. You're only a nurse in the temporary sense of the word. You can go now."

He left.

A cleaner, a woman with whom I'd chatted most days, stuck her head in the door and said, "Hullo." I asked if she knew how to lower the side of the bed and, in a trice, it was done.

I made it back into the moonboot, across to a chair, got dressed and started to pack. Tablet Man came back. I suspect he had worked out that the best outcome, for him, from here, would be if I went home. The heat would all be on me, not on him. He offered to remove the cannula. I accepted and my biggest problem was solved.

I loaded up my bags and shuffled down to the nurses' station, where I asked for a form to sign. One nurse provided the form, while another rang Dr. Heart. I could hear her parroting his ruling that I couldn't leave, as I shuffled off toward the exit.

This is known in the trade as a "Discharge Against Medical Advice"[57] and here was I, once again, failing to make friends and influence people. But I was going home and there is no place like home.

A few weeks later, I went to see Dr. Softly in his rooms. His waiting area has a number of signed photos or posters of the Indian Test Cricket team on the walls, so there was plenty to look at.

We settled into Dr. Softly's office for a long session. It seems my bone marrow is *kaput*, which is only a small step from where I was previously, and I remain in need of regular blood transfusions to stay alive. The other development was that I now had something called *myelodysplastic syndrome* (MDS)[58]. This is a step on the road to developing *acute myeloid leukemia* (AML), a more aggressive form than the *chronic lymphocytic leukaemia* (CLL) which started me on this journey.

Dr. Softly said he would refer me to another Indian doctor who specialises in this area, to see if there was space for me in one of

---

[57] As of December 2017, I have been Discharged Against Medical Advice on ten separate occasions. Not once have any of the threatened consequences come to pass, though I suppose there's always the next time...
[58] **MDS**: Symptoms may include feeling tired, shortness of breath, easy bleeding, or frequent infections. Oh, wait! I had all that already...

the exciting clinical trials being run at the moment. And so one door closed, ahead of a new one opening.

As I got up to leave, I asked Dr. Softly if he had ever seen the 2003 Bollywood movie *Munna Bhai MBBS*[59]? He started laughing and said that, in Bollywood, the rule is: "Leave your brains at the door and have a good time." I couldn't help but think that the same rule often applies in Australia.

---

[59] **Munna Bhai MBBS**: *A gangster takes up the study of medicine to please his father.* (Dr. Softly reminded me of the professor in the story with whom most of the conflict occurs, except Dr. Softly has more hair.) A comedy with heart.

Chapter Twenty-Six

In September 2017, Hospital One relocated to new premises. Very expensive[60] new premises. I made my first visit the week after the place opened, for a blood test. It was huge, it was shiny, and it was crowded with volunteer helpers, rubbernecking gawkers and the occasional patient.

All the odd corners that would have, in the old days, been turned into Staff Only enclaves or mysterious store rooms, were, in this remarkable building, reserved for glass-fronted gardens. Some were small plantings of rock, ground cover and creeper; some were expansive collections of scrap metal "art" and plants; all of them were accessible to bored patients and visitors.

The lost storage space had been relocated underground, where robots provided a discreet in-house delivery service.

Yes, robots.

No, not C-3PO[61], though I asked more than once for an available protocol droid, sometimes for laughs and sometimes in a desperate attempt to communicate with staff members.

The robots in view here are German-made *Automated Guided Vehicles* (AGV), which resemble metal coffins on wheels. The 300kg stainless steel robots move linen, waste, instruments, pharmacy products and patients' meals.

---

[60] Public estimates of the cost of the building have fluctuated over the years, with the current figure sitting around $2.3billion Australian.
[61] Often referred to as Threepio, C-3PO was a bipedal, humanoid protocol droid designed to interact with organics, programmed primarily for etiquette and protocol, and fluent in over six million forms of communication. He developed a fussy and worry-prone personality, but... you know all that.

They drive under trolleys, lift (up to 500kg), then take them to their programmed destination at speeds of up to two metres per second. Built-in sensors are designed to make them stop if they encounter any obstruction.

People like me are never supposed to enter areas populated by the AGVs, so I rely on anecdotes from nurses who will, on the slightest provocation, recount a first- or second-hand encounter with a robot down in the bowels of the building.

There have been stories about AGVs which did not stop when confronted by a cheeky nurse; rumours about nurses attempting to surf on the back of a robot; and stories about AGVs which attempted to travel down stairs, a task for which they are not equipped. I don't know if that was a programming failure or an early sign of artificial intelligence experimenting with independent planning, ahead of a possible invasion of the Sudetenland[62].

In the old days, orderlies used to wheel stuff around. Now robots carry it, but the orderlies have to walk with the robots, just in case.

Robot Walker.

That's a job now. The future arrived early in Adelaide.

During my first transfusion at the new hospital, I coughed and coughed, and sweated heavily, for no apparent reason. This alarmed some of the nurses and they engaged in a rolling whispered conversation, which culminated in a visit from a Haematology intern. She was a tired-looking young woman who had been in the job at this brand-new hospital less than two days. I suspect she was approaching total overload long before she met me.

---

[62] The Nazi seizure of the Sudetenland was an early indication of their plan to conquer the world and enslave the non-Aryan humans. It's not well-known that the Dalek cry of "exterminate, exterminate" dates from this period.

It became obvious early on that her preferred option was to admit me to the hospital. For her: problem solved. For me: the waking nightmare of daily battle with people unable to see past The Rules. I dislike being in hospital. I hate having to explain things to people who are not listening. And I felt I didn't have enough strength left to do battle with entrenched stupidity.

With the benefit of hindsight, the very best thing I could have done was go along with the hospital admission idea.[63] Instead, I gave the young intern enough reason to try the other alternative: blood test, sputum test, and a severe talking-to. She didn't have time to administer the talking-to, so she gave me a piece of paper and delegated the talking-to to a nurse.

The substance of the talking-to was a repetition of The 38 Degree Rule. *If your temperature goes past 38°C, you must get yourself to the Emergency Department, post-haste.*

I had been hearing versions of this rule this since 2007, though it never made much sense to me.

The first thing is, How do you know your temperature has gone past 38°C? That's only possible if you are constantly taking your own temperature.

Seriously? That's what I had to do? Take my temperature every... *what...* ten minutes? For the rest of my life? That wasn't a practical option for me. Unless I was an inpatient and someone else was taking obs at designated intervals.[64]

---

[63] It is not easy for me to admit that I have my own sizeable supply of stupidity. It shows up when I'm tired and grumpy, and takes control. I should never be left in charge of nuclear weapons.

[64] Even that can be a problem, given that so many of the people administering temperature tests lack sensitivity. A series of ungentle entries into the earhole can leave you with a soreness which doesn't heal for weeks. (The worst I ever experienced was at the hand of a G.P. I had to check afterwards to see if he'd drawn blood.) I now insist on administering the test myself.

The second problem was the *Get yourself to the Emergency Department* bit. On the best of days, that would chew up at least an hour. When I finally arrived, would I still be above 38°C, or would my faithless body have reverted to a normal temperature and left me looking a fool?

The question weighed on my mind.

It used to be that I clung to any piece of paper provided by a doctor, especially anything with a doctor's name on it. My theory was that the next person in the chain would be filled with curiosity and seek out whatever information they might be able to glean from a colleague.

I thought that. No one told me that.

Of course, I was wrong.

In this case, the piece of paper I had was a copy of a blood test form. The form had two sets of crossings-out, and the residual data contained an obvious error. I was sick; she was exhausted. I'm not sure which is worse.

And though I attempted to pass the piece of paper to people I later encountered in the Emergency Department, they regarded it with suspicion, as though they saw their peers as competitors and were worried about looking like they were in less than full masterful control of every situation. A fatuous notion, but there it is.

When I arrived the next day for the second unit of blood, I was greeted by the sight of people hastily donning face masks. I heard someone say, "He has influenza type C. It showed up on the sputum test."

That didn't sound good.

I spent the day in a face mask in a single bay, feeling unloved.

That evening, about six p.m., I checked my temperature and *lo, and behold*, there it was: 38.6°C. We got ourselves organised, rang for a taxi and coughed our way back. We were inside the front door of the brand new Emergency Department at about 7:00pm.

This part of the building is designed like an old-fashioned castle, with layers of defenses. The first area held a TRIAGE window, an information desk, some remarkably uncomfortable seats, a cold drinks machine which accepted your money but released no drinks, and more cops and security staff than potential patients.

An E.D. nurse came bounding out, tail wagging, all pleased to see me. He had recognised me from the night of the Queen's Birthday C.C.F. drama and was thrilled with the repeat business. Later, when an Irish doctor rehearsed her understanding of my situation, based on this nurse's report, most of the info related to the June, not the September, event. The E.D. nurse had conflated the two events and coloured his report with the more interesting elements from my previous visit.

We sat on a set of uncomfortable chairs and I coughed. Then we moved to some slightly less uncomfortable chairs and I coughed some more.

A guy from the information desk came over and offered me a face mask. For my comfort, he said, though I suspect it was more for his peace of mind.

For about two hours, I coughed, while my wife tried to coax a drink from the machine. Without success. She wished loudly for the power of the *Fonzie Touch*[65], but that dated from the nineteen-fifties and had no power in this 21st century building.

---

[65] **The Fonzie Touch:** A power, possessed by Arthur Fonzarelli in the TV series *Happy Days*, to make electrical equipment work simply by hitting it. My wife has a habit of striking inanimate objects which displease her by failing to work on command, but has never shown a productive return.

Then we were summoned from the general E.D. waiting area and invited into the assessment area. We collected our goods and chattels, and hobbled inside, only to be stopped by the intern and told to go back, because he had to see "a sick patient" first. That boosted my expectation levels, as I was obviously not sick.

Eventually I rose in the pecking order and we received a second invitation to step inside the Emergency barrier. The red velvet rope was lifted and we entered this exclusive night club on red carpet, to the accompaniment of flashing camera lights, crowd applause, and the press of a bunch of media interviewers. At least, that was the fantasy version.

The reality was more mundane; the rope an electronic door, the flashing lights reflections from a stationary ambulance, the crowd applause echoes of the security team laughing at a policeman's joke, and the crowd a small team in gowns and masks making sure I didn't wander off to more interesting parts of the building.

We were led into a small room with a bed and an uncomfortable chair. In all, I spent twelve hours loitering in the Emergency Department, the first ten of them in company with my wife, until she grew so tired and irritated that she walked out and went home.

It all started well enough; questions from a nurse, followed by questions from the Irish doctor, followed by an awful lot of nothing. This would be shown in an independent film as a scene wherein the actors appear, one on chair, one on bed; jump-cut to the alternate sitting on bed, the second on chair; jump-cut to one pacing aimlessly, while the other looks to be in agonising discomfort on the chair, before moving to the bed for more of the same. A clock in the background would grind out the hours, with the actors wilting visibly, until the point was reached where the interesting-looking female actor leapt to her feet, growled that she had had enough, and disappeared through the curtain.

I was too tired to care. I was hot and covered in sweat. At home, I could stand in front of an electric fan, in a wet T-shirt, and allow the wind-chill to lower my temperature. Not in the hospital. At home I could access an ice-pack from the fridge and move it around strategic spots to ease my discomfort. Not in the hospital. At home, I could get a cold drink whenever I felt like it. Not in the hospital.

They did provide an intravenous antibiotic, which had me tethered to the wall for four hours, and they took a load of blood tests and ECG readings, things I couldn't have done at home.

This night had been the first time I ever heard the phrase *febrile*[66] *neutropenia*[67]. It would not be the last.

In my mind, I set a deadline: by the twelve hour mark, either admit me or tell me to go away. When neither outcome eventuated, I made the decision to leave.

If your temperature goes past 38°C, you must get yourself to the Emergency Department, post-haste. I'd done my part, but encountered a vacuum of intent on the part of the hospital.

When told I was leaving, an offended intern erupted in outrage. He walked with me as I walked out, and made escalating threats as we went. Apparently, I could die at any moment. His final gesture was to ask me what day it was. (If I seemed confused, he had a legal right to restrain me.) I told him the Grand Final[68] wouldn't take place until the following day.

---

[66] **Febrile:** Having or showing the symptoms of a fever.
[67] **Neutropenia:** the presence of abnormally few neutrophils in the blood, leading to increased susceptibility to infection. Neutrophils are a key part of your immune system. They are a type of white blood cell (there are four other types) and make up 55 to 70 percent of your total white cells.
[68] The **Australian Football League Grand Final** is the Superbowl equivalent of Australian sport. It is the biggest event on the calendar and of special interest this year, as The Crows, a local team, would be playing.

I had barely slept in three days. (I have yet to learn how to cough and sleep at the same time.) It was impossible to sleep in the E.D.. Within the hour I was home and fast asleep in my favourite armchair.

Later that day, a doctor rang to tell me that a blood test from last night showed that I had a "blood steam infection" and that I should go back in. I attempted a clarification of what "go back in" might mean in practice. It seems I was being invited to enjoy a rerun of the previous night. I told her that I would rather die than live through a repetition of the E.D. twelve-hour purgatory. I thanked her for her efforts on my behalf and told her I would think about it.

She seemed to be expecting less in the way of verbal gratitude and more in the way of unquestioning obedience, but I had been through that already.

After discussions with my wife, I decided to stay home and try for additional sleep. My understanding of hospital admission techniques was being tested. If I arrived at the E.D. by ambulance, instead of taxi, would I be treated differently? If I arrived early in the day, shortly after the morning shift started and while the place was relatively quiet, instead of at the start of the night shift, would I be seen more quickly?

The next morning we prepared ourselves, then rang for an ambulance. On this, my second visit, I was moved to a room in only six hours.

I viewed these experiences as the cost of purchasing an understanding of hospital dynamics. My conclusion was: If you have a choice in the matter—having made sure your insurance covers it—go the Morning Ambulance route, every time.

And to these questions, I added a firm conclusion: Never go in on Grand Final Day, if a local team was playing. The level of distractedness among staff was extraordinarily high, until it became obvious their team was being thrashed, then the place went quiet and I was transferred to a room.

I was given intravenous antibiotics[69] of various classes, and had blood tests taken every morning. In the wee hours of the seventh day, I asked the night shift nurse about the numbers from the blood tests, with no more in mind than to pass the time. She returned with the information that I had been below the trigger point for a transfusion for at least three days. I spent the rest of the night pondering my situation.

I could only assume that the haematologists had read these test results and were aware that I needed a transfusion, but had chosen to not inform the patient, nor act to achieve a result. This reminded me of the previous year, when a Haematology registrar cancelled a programmed transfusion, without consultation or advice, for her own private amusement. On that occasion, I'd had to voluntarily discharge myself and deal with the Oncology Day Centre as an outpatient, in order to receive the blood I needed to stay alive.

Around 7:00am, I informed the day shift nurse of the situation and advised that, if I didn't receive some firm indication of plans to transfuse me shortly, I would have to discharge myself and go back to the Oncology Day Centre for that service. We heard nothing back, and at 2:30pm, I went home. The Oncology Day Centre booked me in for transfusions on the subsequent Saturday and Monday mornings.

---

[69] **Intravenous antibiotics**: Given the rise of antibiotic-resistant bugs in the world, doctors everywhere are looking for heavier hammers to make their point.

Chapter Twenty-Seven

Three weeks later, I had a bone marrow biopsy at the new hospital. The anaesthetic clinician handling my case was a nervous young woman with an Eastern European accent. At one point she talked about *Stalin*[70]. That bothered me until I worked out that she was probably asking something about *Statin*[71]. Or maybe it *was* Stalin. They'd just made a film about his death. I'm not sure I ever satisfied her on the subject, but I survived the anaesthetic.

The next day, I had an echocardiogram and a chat with my cardiologist. The big news was that I had graduated from *aortic sclerosis*[72] to *aortic stenosis*[73], making me a candidate for a valve replacement. Discussions would take place somewhere in the background, and I would be informed in due course.

On top of all that, I had been enjoying an endless, irritating cough, and the return of a leg infection which had been labelled

---

[70] **Joseph Vissarionovich Stalin** (1878–1953) was dictator of the Soviet Union from the mid-1920s until his death. A paper he wrote titled *Marxism and the National Question* became his most famous work. It was published under the pseudonym of "K. Stalin", a name derived from the Russian word for *steel* (stal). He retained this name for the rest of his life. Stalin was responsible for the deaths of between 20 and 25 million people (including members of my family).
[71] **Statins** are a class of lipid-lowering medications, which have been found to reduce cardiovascular disease and mortality in those who are at high risk.
[72] **Aortic sclerosis** is a mild thickening and mild calcification of the valve. It is commonly encountered on an echocardiogram in patients over the age of fifty.
[73] **Aortic stenosis** (AS) is one of the most common and most serious valve disease problems. AS is a narrowing of the aortic valve opening; it restricts the blood flow from the left ventricle to the aorta and may also affect the pressure in the left atrium. It most commonly develops during aging as calcium or scarring damages the valve and restricts the blood flow. Symptoms may include breathlessness, chest pain (angina), pressure or tightness, fainting, palpitations, a decline in activity level or reduced ability to do normal activities requiring mild exertion, and a heart murmur.

"gravitational eczema" back in 2014. These days it was being referred to as "cellulitis"[74]. I can tell you it was ugly and painful. We tried coating it in Betadine and wrapping it in a bandage. The G.P. prescribed oral antibiotics. Nothing worked.

During a routine visit to monitor progress, the G.P. decided to refer my case to the hospital with a view to them providing intravenous antibiotics. He knows I hate going to the hospital in general and the E.D. in particular, so I called him rude names. He just laughed and said he hadn't seen any photos from the E.D. yet.[75]

I spent most of the next month in hospital, despite my choosing to Discharge Against Medical Advice on three separate occasions.

The first time I arrived at the Emergency Department clutching a letter from my G.P. The doctors there looked at the leg and announced that they weren't going to admit me. I was to be placed in the 'Hospital at Home' program, but first there were some other people who wanted to look at my leg. Vascular and Acute Medical doctors took turns. Some made learned comments. Others took photos.

Once everyone had had their turn, so much time had passed that they'd missed the cut-off point for admitting me to the 'Hospital at Home' program. I would have to stay overnight and be discharged first thing in the morning.

On Thursday, someone discovered complications with the antibiotics; the one being used had a short shelf life, so wasn't

---

[74] **Cellulitis** is a bacterial infection of the skin and tissues beneath the skin. Symptoms and signs of cellulitis include redness, pain and tenderness, swelling, and warmth of the affected area. It can occur anywhere in the body, most frequently on the legs. It is not contagious. Complications include spread of the infection into the bloodstream or to other body tissues. Cellulitis is treated with oral or intravenous antibiotics.

[75] I have been writing him e-mails for a couple of years now, with details of my latest hospitalisation. Those e-mails make up a fair portion of this book. Since we moved to the new building, the e-mails have included photos of that facility.

suitable for suburban use. There was a long Time Out while various experts were consulted. A combination pair of antibiotics, ones with good shelf life, were identified and the program was back on track, but the process had taken so long that I had to stay another night.

By Friday, we discovered that my haemoglobin had dropped to 91. That meant another transfusion, but would I have to self-discharge in order to obtain it as an outpatient? A reluctant consultant eventually approved the transfusion, which took a few hours to organise, then another four hours to administer, by which time I was late to my appointment with the haematologist.

The reason for seeing the haematologist this time was to get the results of the bone marrow biopsy I'd undergone a month earlier. The high point of that meeting came when Dr. Good announced that he could see me living for, oh, another three years.

Meanwhile, I'd lost my place in the 'Hospital at Home' program over the antibiotic confusion. I would have to stay another night and be discharged first thing in the morning.

On Saturday, the cannula they had been using since Wednesday had exceeded its 48 hour limit, so it was removed. The house Jelco Nurse (*yes, they have a full-time cannula nurse!*) was summoned. She was so good, I dubbed her 'OneShot'.

The Saturday lunch arrived and proved to be inedible. A young woman came in and asked about the food. I offered it to her, but she turned her nose up at it, then asked me what I would do. I told her I was going to light a small fire and cook a rabbit, celery and cashew stir-fry, with my secret sauce.

She became agitated. Not at the celery and cashew. Not at the secret sauce. Not even at the thought of the fire. No, she wanted to know about the rabbits. Where would I get them?

That surprised me. She must have passed them a hundred times. I took her for a short walk and showed her a giant mural on a second floor corridor wall. It was of an Australian bush scene: hill, trees, grass. If you looked closely you could see that the staff had added small pictures of rabbits, contrary to all the rules. It seems I'm not the only one who celebrates life with an occasional display of rebellion.

After that, all we had to do was wait for the 'Hospital at Home' supervisor to come at 1:00pm, to approve my inclusion in the program. By 2:00pm he hadn't appeared, so we left.

This bold display impressed the supervisor and we were added to the 'Hospital-at-Home' roster. That worked out to eight home visits—two per day for four days—for eager nurses (and trainees) to administer intravenous antibiotics. Then I was reduced to oral antibiotics, with the same results as last time.

Ten days later, I dropped by for a Group & Match blood test ahead of the next day's transfusion. I was seen by my favourite blood-taking needle jockey, known as " Matron[76]". She ordered me downstairs to the Emergency Department. I was febrile, had been for a couple of days; was coughing like an old steam engine; and generally looked worse than usual.

At TRIAGE, a cheerful E.D. nurse took my temperature, which was—naturally—now normal. I dropped my head in shame, turned, and was about to shuffle off into the hideous glare of day, when she ushered me inside, onto a bed and drew the curtains.

Once inside, I was lost to the system almost immediately, partly because I arrived mid-handover, and partly because I had been filed in one of the noisy containers near the ambulance access doors.

Hours rolled by. Eventually, I heard a thin voice enquiring for me. I bellowed, "Follow the cough!"

---

[76] "Matron" Angela is one of the few in The System in whose judgment I have confidence, despite the way she always laughs at me.

This brought a gallows laugh from the police and security people, and won me promotion to a recognisable assessment stall in a visible traffic-flow neighbourhood, and the tender ministrations of a series of interns. There was the usual maelstrom of questions and confusions. My summary documents helped, they said; even if their minds were more focused on the next case, the one that hadn't arrived yet.

The goal/problem/challenge was to obtain some blood. We were as one on this point. A valiant struggle ensued as intern after heroic intern stepped forward to join battle with the beast and win the heart of the princess.

I was laid back on a bed with eyes closed, enduring the pain and shame as best I've learned how over the years. I failed to recognise then that, not only were they ploughing furrows as they went, but they were too busy or too important to close the minor wounds they left behind. I was bleeding onto my hand / arm / shirt / bed sheet / floor.

Somewhere around then—it was roughly 7:00pm—it all came together. I can't recall the details accurately; please don't quote me. In the midst of coping with the pain of the moment, I released an Anglo-Saxon expletive, a skill I mastered in child-hood. (I was fluent in Housing Commission[77] patois by age seven.) My 'shi-it!' or 'far-ark' or whatever it was, drew a sharp rebuke from a new player, who identified himself as a 'Krensky' or 'Krapsky' or some such, and made it known that he didn't abide expletives from *untermenschen*.

"Don't do it again."

"Really? Far-ark!"

---

[77] **Housing Commission**: *Housing Commission* in the state of Victoria; *Housing Trust* in the state of South Australia; "The Projects" would be the American equivalent.

"Okay, that's it. You're out of here!"

"Shit! See ya later."

Krapsky departed. The other worried-looking intern departed. I moved to a low chair to fix my shoes, and was shocked by all the blood on view. I snapped a quick picture and reflected on the fact that I'd been kicked out of Hospital One, without ever being formally admitted. This was a new low.

I practised deep breathing, while contemplating my options. The last time I'd seen Dr. Good, my treating specialist, he'd been deeply offended that I had become an inpatient without him ever being informed that I was in the building. He was doubly enraged when he attempted to treat me as an outpatient, and issue me some Group & Match forms, while I was an inpatient. The computer told him to bugger off and his blood pressure became visibly elevated.

I rang the switchboard, asked for Dr. Good, and was put through. (I'm still amazed by that.) I explained my situation, and Dr. Good said he would send someone.

Then the worried-looking intern reappeared and started a word game designed to make me say I was happy with things. Mostly I just looked at him, or occasionally made it plain I had accepted the Krapsky Closure. Krapsky had kicked me out. Fair enough. Now we would deal with that fact.

The worried-looking intern did not look comfortable with the situation and tried again. We went round his mulberry bush more times than I can remember, then a Haematology intern arrived.

She took blood, had me bundled up, and I was moved to the fourth floor. Two days later I was moved to the seventh floor. I don't remember much about that time, except I knew my haemoglobin had slid down into the low 70s and no one was doing anything about it. I spent much of one day crying. I was so weak, so tired, and felt entirely helpless. I barely slept in eight days; tiredness covered me like a blanket.

I barely ate[78]. (They block diabetics from ordering real food, as a punishment for being diabetic, substituting instead products that have been stripped of salt, fat, and gluten—everything that makes food *food*—and replaced it with a load of artificial colouring, artificial flavouring, and artificial preservatives, thus turning natural food into a foul-tasting chemical-sodden mass of dubious nutritional value.)

I stopped taking much in the way of insulin, which provoked a fearful response from 'nurses' who lack the mental agility to move past the numbers to the significance of the numbers. If they had controlled my insulin, I would have been dead long ago.

I had a PICC[79] line inserted. This proved to be effective and alleviated the constant fear of being assaulted by incompetent interns hunting for invisible veins. The process of having it installed was reasonably straight forward and, if not actually "painless" as I had been promised, it was a minor discomfort compared to, say, a bone marrow biopsy without anaesthetic.

I had a visit from an Infectious Wounds doctor, a young woman who had a wonderful time peeling away the dead flesh that had accumulated around my leg wound. She said she would be back the next day, but I never saw her again.

There was a Haematology intern whom I called Muppet Boy. I think he was mentally damaged somehow. He would walk up to

---

[78] I lost thirty-six kilos in a few months. My clothes now hang off me. My wife seized on this as an opportunity to go shopping, and kept coming home with clothes that made me look like a schoolboy. I remain convinced that, given time, I'm going to put all the weight back on.

[79] **PICC line.** A *Peripherally Inserted Central Catheter* is a form of intravenous access that can be used for a prolonged period of time.

me and shout into my face. I asked him not to, but he persisted in the practice. At one point he asked to take blood. This worried me. I agreed to give him one shot. He tried and failed. Then he started a second attempt and I rebuffed him. He must have been expecting this, because he pulled out a piece of paper that recorded the fact I had 'refused' a service.

I kept waiting for the transfusion I desperately needed, but nothing happened. I complained to a competent nurse one afternoon and she went to investigate. It turned out that Muppet Boy had been sitting on a release form, just to punish me.

The Group & Match was into the last four hours of its life when they finally set up the transfusion.

When I'd had enough and announced I was leaving the hospital, Muppet Boy was the one they sent to talk me out of it. His offer was basically a payoff in drugs: "What will it take to get you to stay? Pain-killers, sleeping tablets, what would you like? I can get you the strong stuff."

I couldn't get away from him fast enough.

Chapter Twenty-Eight

I developed a painful spot on my backside, a raised one centimetre bump perched on the side of the cliff that leads downward, into the valley of the freckle[80]. Wherever I sat, however I sat, the thing complained. Even lying in bed could be a source of discomfort should the sheets bunch up in the wrong place.

I managed this new problem in a manly fashion: I ignored it and waited for it to go away.

It didn't go away.

I took to administering ointments. There was lanolin, always reliable where gentle soothing is required. There was a modern equivalent of *Preparation H*; more expensive and probably less effective than the original. Then I tried a cortisone ointment. This stuff, I was told, is an amazing healer: You'll be right in no time.

I wasn't right, not even in a long time.

I'm an old ocker[81]. We tend to be gentle, cheerful, helpful fellows. Usually reliable. Not much trouble, given regular feeding; but we have our own taboos, one of which states that it is bad form to stick your arse in other people's faces.

I share the reluctance of my class in this area, and so it was only after weeks of discomfort that I broke down and asked my wife to take a gander.

---

[80] **Freckle** in Australian means "anus".
[81] **Ocker** is both a noun and adjective for an Australian who speaks and acts in a rough and uncultivated manner, while employing a broad Australian accent.

She took a quick squizz[82] and described the problem as an *excoriation*.

"Nothing to worry about."

I have a rule: any physical problem that requires a five syllable name is always something to worry about. Especially if I don't know what the five syllable word means in a given context.

I worried.

The bump went on hurting.

I took to frequent complaining.

My wife relented. She would take another look, this time while wearing her glasses. (I could understand her reluctance: a close study of the hairy orifice requires a dedication beyond the normal course of duty.) Her revised assessment was that this was an abscess[83] and somehow related to the cellulitis; which was, at that time, rampaging about my right leg, and laying waste to all in its path.

And so began a daily program of my bending at the waist, bare arsed, in a posture which never failed to remind me of high school and of my receiving yet another caning at the hands of one of the Marist Brother sadists.

My wife restricted herself to the snapping on of a pair of blue rubber gloves, the Wet Wipe cleansing of the area, and the application of some antiseptic ointment. This was instantly absorbed by my underpants[84] and I worried that the whole thing was a waste of time.

---

[82] **Squizz**: A glance, usually to satisfy personal curiosity. (My wife has an extensive supply of personal curiosity.)
[83] **Abscess**: A skin abscess is a tender mass; usually caused by an infection. Inside, they are full of pus, bacteria and debris.
[84] Yes, Stacey, I was wearing underpants. Thanks for asking.

I would like to say that I dealt with it all in a brave manly fashion, but I felt myself being infantilised. Real men don't have their arses wiped by their wives. Or so I thought.

Then, one morning, we moved past the wipe-and-grease pattern. A sharp, savage pain exploded. My wife muttered that she had wrenched off the outer crust, and was already removing the pus and accumulated contents of the wounded area; an action, she assured me, that was sure to lead to the healing of the abscess.

I restricted myself to sobbing pitifully, while holding on to the arms of the chair I was balanced against.

As my wife predicted, so it came to pass. Over a period of months, as the pain diminished, her frequent comment was that, "It's getting better," until one day it was.

Chapter Twenty-Nine

I was receiving a transfusion in the Oncology Day Centre on Friday December 1, when the nurse started to fret about my leg and called an intern, who worried about my mention of chest pain and decided to move the problem along. Jenny B[85] placed me in a wheelchair, and whisked me to the sixth floor.

My room was the last at the end of a corridor. It had a huge picture window at the end, immediately outside my door. This attracted all sorts, especially as Australia was about to play England at cricket in a Day/Night match, and the hospital had a fair view of Adelaide Oval where the event would take place.

The pig farmers came in on Sunday morning, moved to the window, rang home to the farm and shouted instructions. They worked in relays while I cowered in my room, until about 1:00pm, when they all left for the cricket.

I was placed on eight-hourly Intravenous antibiotics, carefully programmed to include a midnight dose, which guaranteed me little or no sleep.

A couple of mornings later, I was nodding into my bowl of Romanian breakfast cereal (*Guaranteed To Contain No Body Parts*), when an almighty THUMP against the side of the building had me sitting bolt upright. At first I thought a giant wedge-tailed eagle[86] must have crashed into the side of the building, but soon discarded that possibility.

---

[85] **Jenny B**: One of a handful of ninja-grade needle jockeys for whom I have immense respect. She understands the concept of "go the second mile."
[86] The **wedge-tailed eagle** is a large brown bird of prey, the largest in Australia. It has a wingspan up to 2.84 m (9 ft 4 in) and a length up to 1.06 m (3 ft 6 in).

Leaping into action, I sprinted to the window, opened the blind, and met Rusty, my friendly local window cleaner. He was descending from the sky in a metal box, which swung and bounced and banged against the building, leaving Rusty looking totally unperturbed.

The window design in my room was one of several variations on offer in the hospital. It consisted of a large picture window on the left and a smaller, heavily-framed window on the right. This had a built-in winder, which—after an hour of relentless cranking—could open the window far enough to admit air, noise, window cleaner dialogue and, following peak hour (when they parked surplus trains directly below), diesel fumes.

That night, I had an MRI[87]. It was a horrible experience. The machine gave off loud, unpleasant noises. That is to say, LOUD NOISES. They clamped a pair of headphones over my ears, then asked me the fateful question: "Do you like music?" As it happens, I like music and foolishly said so. They asked what I would like to listen to. Before being whisked away into this technological dungeon, I had been listening to Frank Zappa's *Billy the Mountain*[88], and mentioned the fact. They said, "Okay."

Now I know what you're thinking: *That's nice. They'll play the fat guy some music.* That's what I thought. As usual, I was wrong.

For a set of headphones to play music—that's real music, as distinct from noise—it needs to contain wires that can carry an electrical current. Wires like that would be ripped out by the

---

[87] **Magnetic Resonance Imaging** (MRI) is a scanning procedure that uses strong magnets and radiofrequency pulses to generate signals from the body. These are processed by a computer to create images of your insides.
[88] **Billy the Mountain**: a song about a mountain, his wife, and Studebaker Hoch, fantastic new super hero of the current economic slump.
You can never really tell about a guy like that
(Whether he's really a nice person or if he just smiles a lot),
Or if he has a son named 'Pinocchio', or what?
Don't bother, unless you live in L.A. and can tolerate Nixonian-level expletives.

magnets inside an MRI machine and the headphones destroyed. Any head inside the headphones would experience a level of unpleasantness that is scary to imagine.[89]

No, what I heard was a LOUD noise. After some fifteen minutes or so, the noise stopped and a technician told me we were halfway through.

I told her that Frank Zappa must be grateful he's dead, as he was always particular about the sound quality of his music. She explained about the wires and said this noise was being transmitted by air. How that works I have no idea, but I begged for mercy and she turned off the noise of the head-phones, leaving only the noise of the MRI. It was a thirty minute procedure, but I felt as though I were inside the machine for a full three weeks. And they were not a nice three weeks.

As 2017 drew to a close, I began receiving home visits from the RDNS[90]. At first, they cleaned up the PICC line and did some tidy up work on the leg infection. As we approached the holidays[91], my transfusions were passed to the RDNS as well. The workload for the Oncology Day Centre became impossible, but—as usual—they found a way. My admiration for that team grew greater still.

December 2017 started well, then things fell apart. I remember almost nothing of Boxing Day[92], other than occasionally seeing my wife looking at me and saying things like, "You're acting strangely."

---

[89] There is a video on YouTube from UC Berkeley, which demonstrates what happens to metal in an MRI.
[90] The **Royal District Nursing Service** is a not-for-profit community health and care provider in Adelaide. It is known as "RDNS" in South Australia and "Silver Chain" throughout the rest of Australia.
[91] **The holidays**: Fewer working days, fewer staff on duty, but the same number of patients requiring tranfusions, chemotherapy infusions, etc.
[92] **Boxing Day** is a holiday celebrated the day after Christmas Day. It originated in the UK and is celebrated in a number of other countries. Also known as the second day of Christmastide, and Saint Stephen's Day.

From my point of view, I was aware of falling asleep frequently. A couple of times, I woke out of a deep sleep, with a hyper-urgent need to urinate. And apparently I did just that, while standing on the carpet in the middle of the lounge room.

My wife called for an ambulance. When we arrived at the hospital, my temperature was 40°C. Staff were quick to put me in incontinence pants, in the hope of reducing the scale of the cleaning task.

The next few days were spent in the fog of a fever-driven nightmare. Giant, mucous-coated pigs followed me about[93], watching, waiting, and sneering at my helplessness. These hallucinations were worse than any I experienced when eating magic mushrooms[94] back in the 1970s.

The next few weeks were filled with round-the-clock intravenous delivery of antibiotics and platelets, and sundry other things. My temperature ranged from 34.7° to 40°C. The culprit was a wee beast called *pseudomonas*[95], which had gotten into my blood somehow.

I developed gastritis, which bothered me for weeks. No one could work out the cause of that. I was prodded, pressed and poked by a range of specialists. My gall bladder was made chief suspect for quite a while, but no consensus formed. They solved the problem by no longer asking the question.

---

[93] I was lying in a hospital bed, not going anywhere; but hallucinations being what they are, I was convinced I was walking around some Spanish-style piazza.
[94] **Magic mushrooms** come in a range of classes. The ones I experimented with were called *gold tops*; they contained *psilocybin*, grew in cow pats on the northern New South Wales coast and tasted foul. Though I have seen *amanita muscaria* mushrooms (of *Alice in Wonderland* fame) growing in the Adelaide hills, I have never tried them. Note: I do not recommend you try them. They are not a doorway to spiritual insight and can leave you seriously damaged.
[95] **Pseudomonas** infections are caused by a bacteria found widely in the environment. Infections can occur in any part of the body, but a blood infection is one of the most severe. Symptoms may include fever, chills, fatigue, and muscle and joint pain.

Once they stopped the I/V antibiotics, I couldn't see the point of staying in hospital. After twenty-two days, I announced that I was going home. They didn't like it, but the doctors had seen enough to take me seriously and they worked with me. I was formally discharged. and given a bunch of prescriptions and RDNS referrals.

Chapter Thirty

Meanwhile, Dr. Good had a plan to treat the MDS by placing me on a drug called *Azacitidine*[96], but I wasn't well enough to cope with the potential side effects[97].

First, I needed a course of something called *Filgrastim*[98]. Naturally, Filgrastim has its own list of side effects: Pain in the left upper part of the stomach or the tip of the left shoulder, fever, shortness of breath, trouble breathing, fast breathing, wheezing, dizziness, sweating, hives, rash, itching, swelling around the mouth, face, eyes, stomach, feet, ankles, or lower legs, unusual bruising or purple markings under the skin, unusual bleeding or bruising, nosebleeds, decreased urination, and tiredness. I only developed twelve of these.

---

[96] **Azacitidine** is an anti-cancer chemotherapy drug, classified as an "antimetabolite" and a "demethylation" agent. It is used in the treatment of myelodysplastic syndrome (MDS) and chronic myelomonocytic leukemia (CMML).
Methylation of DNA is a major mechanism that regulates gene expression in cells. An increase in DNA methylation can result in the blockage of the activity of "suppressor genes" that regulate cell division and growth. When suppressor genes are blocked, cell division becomes unregulated, allowing or promoting cancer. Demethylation restores normal function to the tumor suppressor gene. *Antimetabolites* are very similar to normal substances within the cell. When the cells incorporate these into the cellular metabolism, they produce a direct cytotoxic effect that causes death of rapidly dividing cancer cells.
[97] The following **side effects** can occur for patients taking *azacitidine*:
Nausea, low red blood cell count, low platelet count, vomiting, fever, low white blood cell count, diarrhoea, fatigue, injection site redness, constipation, ecchymosis, petechiae, cough, shortness of breath, weakness, chills, injection site pain, joint and muscle pain, headache, poor appetite, sore throat, back pain, confusion, dizziness, swelling in ankles, chest pain, nosebleed, weight loss, abdominal pain, rash, anxiety, low potassium, upper respiratory infection, itching, depression, and insomnia.
[98] **Filgrastim** is used to decrease the chance of infection in people with certain types of cancer. It helps the body make more neutrophils.

And so, here we are: not quite in the pink[99], but looking forward to better days ahead. 2018 is full of promise.

The Charcot foot has settled down. I've had new orthotics made and am presently on the hunt for a non-pair of shoes, ones which will accommodate a wide left foot and a normal right foot. As mementos of that particular adventure, there is a corner of my bedroom wherein stand a pair of crutches, a short moonboot, a long moonboot, and a CROW boot.

The aortic valve replacement remains a question for the future.

I'm still having regular transfusions, but usually at home, thanks to RDNS. Now I can watch a favourite movie while waiting for the long, slow process to end. The bonus is that I get to introduce great movies to young people who had never heard of them.

Thank you for your patience, Gentle Reader. My life is filled with excitement. I hope your's is as well. Enjoy the *Lessons Learned* in the next chapter. And, as my in-laws are wont to say: Keep yourself nice.

---

[99] **In the pink:** The general usage of this phrase has altered somewhat since it first entered the language. These days, it has the specific meaning of 'the pink of condition', that is, in the best possible health. In the earliest citations of 'in the pink', the meaning was 'the very pinnacle of something', but not necessarily limited to health. There is an early example in Shakespeare's *Romeo & Juliet*, 1597.

Chapter Thirty-One

Some readers of the first edition demanded "a moral to the story". That had me thinking for a while; eventually I came up with the following *Lessons Learned*.

LESSON ONE. *Take photos.*

In those depressed times, when the whole world looks dark and desperate, photos can be useful for reminding you of how far you've come. They are also useful for letting others know how much you've been suffering. Bruises heal up more quickly than you expect; the evidence fades swiftly. Be prepared with happy snaps so you can commemorate your times of torment and celebrate your recovery.

LESSON TWO. *Write notes for yourself.*

It's your body, it's your life: you're responsible.

Sure, there are countless caring, hardworking doctors and nurses on the job, but you are just one of hundreds of patients they will be seeing over a short period. They mean well, most of them, but they are under pressure. I couldn't tell you how many times doctors or nurses said they were going to do something and never did, distracted as they were by the pressures of the day. A simple thing like a change of shift can disconnect you from promises made, never mind having your doctor go off on holidays.

I learned to handle this by writing notes. About everything. My wife kept a version also, which proved helpful with regard to the times when I was too sick to keep track of things.

LESSON THREE. *Ask*.

You're desperate to sit up comfortably but there's no chair in your room? Ask for one. No rubbish bin for you to put all those tissues you're using to cope with a slow nose bleed? Ask. You'll be amazed at what they have stashed away in cupboards or spare rooms in a large hospital.

LESSON FOUR. *Complain*.

Don't be a troublemaker, but don't suffer in silence either. Many simple problems can be resolved by bringing a problem to the attention of someone up the line.

I took it as far as writing to the Minister for Health on a couple of occasions, when I had serious concerns about things that had been happening or not happening to me. The sudden improvements in my treatment were striking.

LESSON FIVE. *Be aware of potential conflict between the experts*.

Different areas in the same hospital can have conflicting views on your treatment.

The view of the Haematology Unit as to what constituted a reasonable level of haemoglobin for someone like me was in vivid contrast with the view held within the Oncology Unit. Put bluntly, the Oncology people understood the impact of the loss of bone marrow functionality, while the lower level Haematology people did not. This lead to transfusions I needed being cancelled, and to the one time I became seriously angry and rattled my cage. In the end, I received what I needed.

I was given conflicting advice by a vascular surgeon and an orthopaedic surgeon. One wanted for me to exercise, to keep the blood moving; the other wanted me to immobilise that leg. The orthopaedic surgeon won out, and I was fast-tracked to a CROW boot, which allowed me to walk safely.

If you find yourself caught between two areas of the hospital, refer to Lesson Four.

LESSON SIX. *Be prepared*.

I keep a bag packed and ready to go, one that contains the things I need or want for a sense of personal comfort. Like an iPod with headphones, for the miserable midnight hours spent in sleepless discomfort. Don't say to yourself, *I'll remember when the time comes*. No, you won't. There'll be so many other pressures that you'll forget the one thing you most meant to take with you. Be prepared.

LESSON SEVEN. *Go in early*.

For routine procedures, like chemotherapy or transfusions, I always turn up at least thirty minutes early. Yes, I know they have a roster and you've been given a strict time for when they can see you, but stuff happens. Some patients arrive late, others don't arrive at all. By simply being available, you're doing the staff a favour. The sooner they get started, the sooner they get finished. They have homes to go to, families to care for. Be a friend and be early. The worst thing that can happen is that you get to read the book you took in with you.

LESSON EIGHT. *Be grateful*.

I know I've focussed in this book on the bad and the sad, but that's the nature of creating interesting reading. In reality, I am deeply grateful for all the care I have received from many wonderful people. I'm always saying, "Thank you," and sometimes I buy them chocolate. Nice chocolate, like the type you'd buy your Mum. To make up for forgetting her birthday.

LESSON NINE. *Be cheerful.*

Keep your sense of humour.

I copped a lot of flak, and even lost a friend, for saying that I'd written a funny book about going through treatment for cancer.

"There's nothing funny about chemotherapy," I was told.

At one level that's true, and I have spent more than a few miserable hours trapped in a chair with a drip in my arm, but I believe that if you look for the funny side of life, you'll find it.

LESSON TEN. *Stand up for yourself.*

You will meet a lot of nice, friendly, caring people in hospitals. You will also meet a few lazy, selfish, nasty, bullying types. Don't be intimidated. If it sounds wrong, challenge it. Ask to speak to their supervisor. Ask to speak to a doctor. Don't accept medication just because a nurse is handing it around. Don't allow just anyone to inject you with insulin or other drugs. Be sure it's right for you. Stand up for yourself.

LESSON ELEVEN. *Practice humility.*

When in hospital, it's nice to chat with a specialist occasionally. The centre-of-attention feeling generated by the solicitous-looking entourage can boost your confidence for a moment or so, but the really important people in hospitals are the "menials". The person who empties the bin, or cleans the toilet[100], or brings your meals, or sweeps the floor, or wheels your bed to the CT scanner, or cleans the windows: these guys have the real power to make your stay more or less pleasant. Take an interest, be nice to them, learn their names. You won't regret the effort.

---

[100] You'll understand this more fully the first time you suffer explosive diarrhoea. Trust me.

LESSON TWELVE. *For diabetics.*[101]

I know from discussions with other diabetics that the question of who controls the insulin pen can be a major source of drama in hospital.

This is not intended to offend anyone, but... I have to say — purely from my experience in Adelaide — that the average Registered Nurse here has limited insight into the management of diabetes. They know that insulin is involved, and maybe drugs such as metformin/diaformin, but not much more.

My first test of their capacity to manage diabetes comes when I'm admitted to hospital. Do they ask the single most important question, the one every diabetic should be asked at this stage: *When did you last eat?*

The point being that the patient might be on the verge of a hypo. Nursing staff should be ready for that. In a dozen or more hospital admissions I have never been asked that question, not even once. Which meant that I knew from the outset that I would be the one managing my diabetes.

In my early days, I simply refused to do what so many nurses have demanded, i.e., hand over the pen. Later on, I learned to walk the nurse through a series of questions.

a) What do you plan to do with the pen?
This always draws an answer involving their intention to inject me with insulin.

b) How much insulin do you plan to give me?
They usually pluck at the last number they heard I'd taken. (If they have to ask you to provide a number, why are they getting involved?)

---

[101] All the comments that follow presuppose that the patient is *compos mentis* and physically capable of looking after themselves.

c) How do you know I need that much?
They don't. Even the most arrogant begin to falter around here. I provide the helpful hint that there are seven factors[102] I take into account in making that assessment, and ask them what they are. They might guess one or two, but that's it.

d) Are you aware that there was a court case in Australia in 2016 in which a nurse was charged with murdering patients by giving them insulin they didn't need?
Megan Haines, in Ballina, NSW. She was found guilty and sentenced to thirty-six years in prison. (This piece of information alters the emotional context of the conflict. Why are they so eager to put their hands on my insulin?)

e) I like to make the point that I don't have an insulin problem, I have a diabetes problem. Insulin is merely a subset of the available management techniques. Then I ask, Who has overall medical responsibility for the management of my diabetes?
They have no idea, but will guess at various medical officers, never correctly. I tell them it is my endocrinologist, then ask, Who is he? and What was the last instruction he gave concerning the management of my diabetes?

They don't know who he is, so they can't have consulted with him. They don't know what instructions he gave, so how can they comply with them? In other words, there is no medical basis to their plan for an insulin assault on me. Are we back with Megan Haines here? (It is sometimes helpful to ask to see their supervisor about this time, and walk them through the same questions.)

---

[102] Food eaten, exercise undertaken, diabetes medication taken, current BGL, the trend of my BGL (toward hypo- or hyperglycaemia), any alcohol consumed, the impact of other medication (such as steroids like Prednisolone or oral chemotherapy drugs). Other factors can include my emotional state and/or illness.

f) If you're still having trouble, ask the nurses to show you a written instruction from a doctor, authorising them to interfere with the management of your insulin.

There won't be one, not anywhere on your file. Doctors aren't that stupid. And again we find there is no legal or medical justification for their interfering with your insulin.

g) It should never come to this, but, in the most extreme cases, you take them literally. "It's a rule of this ward that patients hand over their insulin pen." Fine, but as you have no intention of handing the pen over, their rule means that you have to leave the hospital.

They will try to call this a Discharge Against Medical Advice, but you insist: No, it's not my choice, That Nurse (*make a note of their name*) has ordered me out. He/she is the one responsible. Oh, and I'll be complaining in writing to the appropriate authorities... *Don't worry. Someone further up the line will jump in and apply a new interpretation of the infamous rule, and you will be left in peace for the duration of your stay.*

Sometimes the road to Person Centred Care involves you standing up for yourself.

LESSON THIRTEEN. *People with faith do better than people without.*

I know that statement will offend some readers, but it can't be helped. It is the truth as I know it. I've been able to see the funny side of my experiences only because I have faith in something — *Someone* — larger than myself.

I'm not preaching here, but I can't ignore the fact that my faith gives me strength to cope with all the things I can't understand and don't enjoy. In time, it will all work out.

His eye is on the sparrow and I know He watches over me.

INDEX

38 Degree Rule 171
A.P.O 150
abscess 188, 189
acute myeloid leukemia 167
acute pulmonary oedema..... 150
Adelaide Oval 191
ailments 104
air biscuit 122
Alien 102
ambulance 87, 89, 104, 109
   159, 174, 176, 182, 194
AML 167
amphetamines 44, 46
anaesthesiologist 28
anaesthetic clinician 30, 179
anaesthetist 28, 30, 31
angiogram 123, 131, 132
Anglo-Saxon 92, 183
animal sacrifices 188
antibiotics 83, 88, 158,
   177, 180, 181, 182, 190, 191,
   194, 195
aortic sclerosis 179
aortic stenosis 179
aortic valve replacement 179,
   198
Apollo 13 24
apple and cinnamon cake 123
arm-wrestling 124
arrhythmia 149
Arrogant Shift Coordinator 88
arthritis 103, 143
artificial intelligence 170
asphyxiate 109
asshole 90
asthma 103, 117, 149

Attila the Hun 109
auctioneer 122
Australian 13, 14, 17, 123, 183
Automated Guided Vehicles 169
autonomic neuropathy 103
Awkward Old Bastard 69
AWOL 87
axilla 157
Azacitidine 197

baby octopus 126, 127
back pain 103
baguette 134
balls 50, 110, 154
bamboo 110, 111
barbecued lip 75
barium swallow 17
Big Hospital Attitude ... 32, 42, 70
Billy the Mountain 192
black turds 48, 49, 50 54
bladder problems 103
bleeding from the eyes 89
Blood Book 53, 83, 113, 114,
   125
blood glucose reading 57, 65
blood pressure 63, 103, 150,
   184
Blood Supply, Wizard Unit ... 115
blood test 40, 47, 48, 53,
   60, 63, 65, 72, 82, 83, 113,
   114, 121, 162, 165, 134, 162,
   165, 169, 171, 172, 175, 176,
   177, 182
blood-soaked concrete 47, 53
blowing off 123
blubber 23
bone marrow biopsy .. 17, 19, 21,
   25, 27, 30, 31, 32, 35, 81, 82,
   158, 164, 165, 179, 181, 185
bone marrow 46, 81, 82,
   167, 200

box of tissues 59, 87
Boxing Day 193
Boxing Tent 95
Boy Scout 49, 109
breathing 109, 110, 122, 149, 150, 151, 184, 197
Bright Young 57, 58, 59
broom closet 21, 117, 119
bus 45
butt-clenching 98

C.C.F. 121, 149, 162, 173
cancer 13, 73, 107, 109, 202
cannula 44, 50, 59, 88, 113, 125, 150, 153, 165, 166, 167, 181
cape 108
cardiologist 123, 130, 131, 153, 158, 179
Carla 135, 138, 139
cartilage 109
cast 118, 138, 139, 143, 144, 145, 146, 147
castor oil 37, 45
CAT scan 21
Catastrophe and Woe 38, 43
catheter 151, 159
Catholic education 49
cellularity 81
cellulitis 180, 188
Charcot arthropathy 133
Charcot foot 103, 138, 142, 147, 198
Charcot Restraint Orthotic Walker 145
Charcot, Monsieur 133
Chatter, Cathy 136, 137, 138, 139, 140
chemotherapy 13, 17, 18, 19, 21, 32. 37, 38, 40, 42, 43, 47, 54, 87, 107, 158, 201, 202

cherry-picker 100
chest x-ray 83, 121, 150
China Doll 21, 22, 24, 25
Chinese banquet 126
chocolate 55, 63, 64, 201
choir invisible 18
chronic lymphocytic leukaemia 167
citizen engagement 28
Cleese, John 19
clench 45, 98
clinical trial 168
clipboards 99
CLL 167
Clockwork Puppy 69, 70, 71
clot 102, 127, 131, 134
Coco Chanel 142
Cold Heart 118, 119
cold sore 73
cold tap 160, 161, 163
comfort station 141
complicated double fold 68
condom 90, 92
confrontation 122
Congestive Cardiac Failure .. 121, 149
constipation 45, 103
consumer engagement 28, 33
Continuous Positive Airways Pressure 150
cortisone ointment 187
costume 108, 128
cough 17, 18, 19, 21, 31, 35, 36, 37, 57, 83, 110, 117, 118, 119, 170. 173, 162, 163, 176, 179, 182
CPAP mask 150
Crimean War 97
CROW boot ... 145, 147, 198, 201
CT scan 19, 21, 74, 117, 158, 162, 162

CT scanner 21, 74, 202
curried egg sandwich.... 122, 123
cynic 28, 47

Dalek 67, 68
Darth Vader 150, 151, 155
day surgery 107
Death Valley........................ 110
debt collector...................... 142
dental hygienist................ 36, 37
dermatologist........................ 73
designer labels 145
diabetes 103, 130, 142, 203, 204
diabetic.......... 28, 30, 55, 57, 58,
  122, 123, 133, 135, 185, 203
diaformin 203
dignity.......................... 119, 124
Discharge Against Medical
  Advice 157, 167, 180, 205
dismount technique 119
diuretic 125, 127, 150
doctor speech 92
dog 38, 66, 94, 115, 123, 126
doubts 146
Dr. Crusty.............. 142, 143, 145
Dr. Dreadful 49, 50, 60, 65, 71
Dr. Good 63, 64, 71, 72,
  181, 184, 197
Dr. Heart 158, 162, 165, 167
Dr. Laser.......................... 74, 75
Dr. Le 30, 31
Dr. Pfhgumbumble 137
Dr. Softly 162, 165, 167, 168
Dr. Strange............................ 73
Dr. Tease............. 19, 32, 35, 36,
  37, 45, 81, 82, 46, 60, 82, 83,
  117, 125, 141
drip 24, 25, 35, 36, 45, 50,
  51, 63, 66, 71, 98, 202
duct tape 24, 27, 110, 111,
  16, 154

dunny.................................... 98
E.C.G. 121, 123, 126, 134, 150
E.N.T. Registrar................94, 99
E.N.T. 90
E.T. the Extra-Terrestrial 153
ears........................ 67, 89, 192
Easter.......... 63, 65, 72, 121, 179
Easter Uprising 63
Eastwood, Clint..................... 87
ebony................................... 98
echocardiogram 123, 124,
  132, 179
eczema....................... 103, 180
electrocardiogram 121
eleven 66, 93, 141
Emergency Department...47, 53,
  54, 58, 63, 83, 87, 88, 89, 91,
  94, 101, 121, 125, 134, 149,
  150, 154, 171, 172, 173, 174,
  175, 180
endocrinologist...............57, 204
endoscopy............................ 50
England 17,18, 19
epistaxis 89, 99, 100, 110
excessive tiredness 121
expletive 92, 151, 183
Exsultate justi 114
eyeball 109, 110
eyes 22, 23, 38, 40, 49, 55,
  76, 77, 78, 89, 92, 104, 110,
  111, 136, 151, 165, 183, 197

Fairbanks, Douglas............... 107
farmers 126, 191
farting 123
febrile neutropenia.......175, 182
fencing 107
fibre-optic cable 101
file................ 29, 33, 90, 93, 127,
  129, 136, 166, 182, 205

Filgrastim 197
Final Insult 151, 158
firing chamber 97
fish 84, 122, 202
five tones 110
fixed smiles 99
flaming torches 40
flatulence 45
flesh-eating crabs 146
flu shot 1212, 124
flunky 98
Flynn, Errol 107
Fonzie Touch 173
food 57, 121, 122, 124,
 125, 126, 163, 166, 181, 185
footnote 14
forest 146
fork 126
formal complaint 29
Frank Zappa 192, 193
freckle 187
frusemide 127
funeral 104
furosemide 127

Gangly Intern 100, 101, 102
gardens 169
gastritis 194
gauze 110
General Practitioner 17, 73
German 117, 169
Get Shorty 89
glasses 77, 79, 80, 188
gloves 93, 188
glowing mice 108
glucose 56, 57, 65
glycaemic irresponsiblity 66
goat-herders 109
Gotcha! 65
Grand Final Day 176
gravitational eczema 103, 180

Group & Match 83, 113, 125,
 182, 184, 186
gweilo 126

haematemesis 11, 13, 14, 15
haematologist 19, 49, 54,
 158, 162, 177, 181
Haematology Registrar ... 85, 177
Haematology Unit 84, 200
haemoglobin 48, 53, 55,
 63, 71, 72, 82, 83, 103, 114,
 125, 165, 181, 184, 200
Haines, Megan 204
hair loss 38
hair removal 146
Hallelujah Chorus 49
healing shoe 143
heart attack, imaginary 131
heart attack, secret 123, 131,
heartburn 103
Heat Shrink plastic 109
heist movie 101
helicopter 125
High Dependency 150
high-five 93
hillbilly 95
hillbilly heroin 105
home 15. 30, 36, 39, 45,
 51, 57, 58, 63, 71, 72, 79, 105,
 111, 115, 124, 127, 132, 135,
 149, 155, 157, 159, 161, 167,
 174, 175, 176, 177, 180, 181,
 182, 191, 193, 195, 198, 201
homeless refuge 111
Homer Simpson 23, 55
Hopoate, John 58
Hospital at Home .. 180, 181, 182
Hospital One 142, 169, 184
Hospital Two 141
Hospital Three 159, 165
hot tap 160

Hungry Jack's 163, 164
hyperspace 23, 110
hypoglycaemia 56, 57, 58, 121, 134

Indian Test Cricket Team 167
Infectious Wounds 185
influenza type C 172
Insyte 44
insulin 28, 30, 57, 58, 64, 65, 69, 70, 71, 28, 129, 153, 185, 202, 203, 204
insulin pen 129, 203, 205
Intensive Care Unit 150
intern 85, 89, 99, 100, 170, 171, 174, 175, 183, 185, 191
intravenous antibiotic 83, 88, 175, 177, 180, 182, 191
Irritated Nurse 68

Jay 92, 93, 94, 101
Jelco 44
Jenny B 114, 191
jiggling 108, 109, 124
Jocks 67, 98,

Karen 90, 93
Kelly, Gene 119
kimchi 126
Kiosk 122, 123
knife 64, 73, 107, 108, 110
Korean 126, 127
Kreemorian Fangor Beast 103
Krusty the Clown 101
Kwang 126, 127
Kylie 36, 37

lanolin 187
Large Bully 59, 60
laser surgery 74
Lasix 127

Laughing Man 160
leeches 17, 146
lettuce 126, 134
leukaemia 4, 17, 21, 35, 36, 81, 108, 158, 167
light source 102
light-thingy 94
lion-tamer 102
lipstick 143
liquid solvent 101
locomotive 108
lunch box 123
lymph nodes 35

machine operator 109
magic mushrooms 194
Magnetic Resonance Imaging 192, 193
Malaysia 126
Mandy Patinkin 107
manly expression 119
mano e mano 94
Maori mask 112
Marist Brothers 49, 188
marmalade 58, 71
Matron 182
Matterhorn 81
McGregor, Ewan 98
MDS 167, 197
Megan Haines 204
Melanie 133, 134, 135, 142, 147
Men in Black 93, 94
menials 48, 202
metformin 203
mice 108
Millenium Falcon 22
missile 97
mood 92
moonboot 135, 144, 163, 166, 198

motto 33, 119, 121
mouse parties 108
MRI 192, 193
Multi-Disciplinary Foot
  Clinic 136
Munna Bhai MBBS 168
Muppet Boy 185, 186
muscle spasm...................... 118
myelodysplastic syndrome .. 103, 167
nausea 39, 40, 103
nebuliser.............................. 121
needle jockey............ 41, 42, 44, 87, 88, 113, 162, 182
needles 20, 24, 38, 40, 41, 87, 150
Neulasta................................ 46
neurologist........................... 133
neuropathy 103, 130, 133
nexus 60
ninja-grade............................ 87
nightmare 171, 194
non-weight bearing.............. 143
North Korea 126
nose bleeds............... 13, 46, 48, 50, 53, 103, 110
nose-breathing..................... 110
nostril grip 87
nostrils 95, 109, 111
nostrovia.............................. 112
noxious gas 122

O&P 138, 139, 143, 147
obs................................ 72, 171
oncologist 19, 20, 28, 35, 47, 60, 127
Oncology Day Centre....... 83, 84, 113, 136, 166, 175, 191, 193
Oncology Unit 84, 200
octopus...................... 126, 127
open space................... 94, 109

opiate withdrawal 105
optometrist 77, 78, 80
Orthotics and Prosthetics.... 138, 143
Overbearing 57, 58, 59
oxycodone.......................... 105
oxygen 126, 149, 150, 153

paedophiles........................... 50
pain relief......... 88, 93, 104, 105
pain.......... 15, 27, 38, 49, 56, 74, 79, 88, 90, 92, 94, 103, 104, 105, 109, 110, 123, 134, 152, 154, 159, 180, 183, 185, 186, 187, 191, 197189,
panic 51, 57, 102, 109, 146
parrot................................... 94
patient participation............. 28
patient-centred care......... 28, 42
Patinkin, Mandy 107
Person-Centred Care 28, 64
pharmacopeia 37, 44
photo 4, 32, 76, 113, 167, 180, 199
PICC line 193
pitchforks 40
pixie dust............................. 113
Pizza Hut 22, 162
plaster cast.... 138, 143, 144, 145
plastic surgeon 48, 107
platelets 88, 194
plumber's tools 101, 102
pneumonia........................... 83
Political Correctness
  Committee...................... 154
Pommy................................. 17
pong................................... 145
potassium............................. 88
Preparation H..................... 187
Prince Phillip........................ 18
prison.......... 50, 54, 78, 130, 204

pseudomonas 194
psychiatrist 17
pulse oximeter 150, 153

Queen's Birthday 149, 173
Queen Elizabeth 17, 18

radiation 108, 109, 110, 111,
radiation commandos 108, 110, 111
rabbit 181, 182
radiotherapy 13, 107, 108
railway track 107
Rainee 11
Rapid Rhino 90, 91, 92, 93, 99, 100, 101
RDNS 193, 195, 198
recreational beard fondler 36
Red Rover 109
remission 17
robots 169, 170
Romeo & Juliet 194
Royal Commission 49
rugby scrum 122
Rule of 80 55
rumpy-pumpy 107
Russian mafia 112

salad roll 53, 57, 122
saline drip 63
saliva 110
schoolboy 75, 99
screaming 88, 98
secret heart attack 123, 131,
shoe-able 143, 147
shopping bags 145
shortness of breath 121, 167, 197
Shoving Woman 77
shower 72, 145, 146, 154, 159, 160, 161, 162, 164

shrieking Dalek 67, 68
side effects 38, 197,
sinusitis 103
skeleton staff 114
skin cancer 107
skittish patients 108
slab-of-meat 84, 88
slinky 119
Stalin 179
Slothful-from-Haematology
 .... 31, 32
Smoker Nurse 64, 65, 66
Smug Nurse 103, 104
Spielberg, Steven 110
Spinal Tap 93
spiritual advisor 19
spring rolls 125
squamous cell carcinoma 107
Stacey 114, 188
stainless steel 27, 38, 48, 102, 169
Star Trek 22
stethoscope 83
street cred 93
street theatre 51
Sudetenland 170
super-powers 108, 109
Surgical Admission Suite 31
swallowing 103, 110
swearing 67, 91, 92, 101
syphilis 142
Syrian gas party 123

Tablet Man 165, 166
tailgate 89
Talking Pillow 99
tall buildings 108
temperature 160, 161, 171, 172, 173, 175, 182, 194
The Rules 54, 57, 58, 59, 64, 69, 171, 182

The System 31, 54, 59, 114, 158, 182,
theatre sister 29
tiger snakes 146
Tiller, Annette 7
toilet 39, 40, 72, 75, 94, 97, 98, 159, 160, 161, 202
total contact cast 144
Trainspotting 98
tramp steamer 122
transfusion 11, 48, 49, 53, 63, 71, 72, 81, 83, 84, 87, 88, 113, 125, 136, 149, 158, 165, 167, 170, 177, 181, 182, 186, 191, 193, 200, 201198,
Triage 53, 63, 73, 82
trichotillomania 36
trivia 104
troponin 123, 131
Tufnel, Nigel 93
Twilight Zone 113

ugly swollen ankles 121
ultrasound 88, 134,

vacuum 22, 74, 150, 152, 175
valve replacement 179, 198
Vaseline 110
Viet Nam 142
vomit 9, 15, 88

waiter 126, 127
walrus 110
waltz 27, 151, 152
Waterproof Leg Protectors .. 146
wedge-tailed eagle 191
weights 110, 111
white cells 45
white dress 49
white handkerchief 99
wide, brown land 126
wife 11, 15, 18, 29, 44, 48, 51, 55, 59, 60, 63, 67, 71, 84, 88, 128, 141, 144, 156, 163, 173, 174, 176, 187, 188, 189, 193, 194, 199
Wifely 11
wimp 20
window cleaner 192
Witness Protection 24
wobbly member ... 134, 151, 152
wombat-fighting 124
Wookie 22, 25
work colleagues 38
wuss 89

YouTube 91

Zappa, Frank 192, 193
Zimm, Harry 89

Books by Henry G. Sheppard

The Evidence, 1995, ISBN 1-876126-15-9
Currently out of print.

Play the Devil, 2013, ISBN 9-781477-537466

Haematemesis, Expanded 3rd Edition, 2018,
ISBN 10-1986007421   ISBN 13-9781986007429

www.ingramcontent.com/pod-product-compliance
Lightning Source LLC
Chambersburg PA
CBHW052249220526
45471CB00001B/255